Optavia Air Fryer Cookbook

Cook and Taste 150+ Healthy Lean & Green Meals, Burn Fat without Feeling Hungry and Be Super Energetic

By

Rosa Murphy

Rosa Murphy

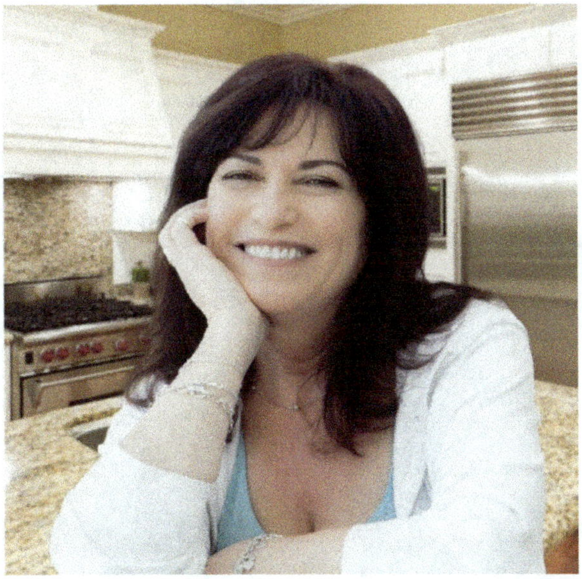

"Happiness is homemade"

Rosa Murphy is a 50-year-old woman, a mother of three girls and a great chef. She is also a fantastic writer and has written more than 20 books regarding different diets to help people. She is an experienced nutritionist and chef. She also give lectures about health and nutrition in Universities.

Her passion for becoming an outstanding chef one day made her travel worldwide, where she worked in different kinds of restaurants.

Speaking of experience, Rosa started her chef career in Los Angeles when she was just 23 years old. After she worked as a chef in different restaurants worldwide for about ten years. Four years in Sidney, three in Japan and around three years between Monte Carlo, Italy and London.

Besides all this, Rosa also teaches kids how to cook whenever she is free to do so

Table of Contents

Introduction

Optavia is a weight reduction or maintenance strategy that recommends eating a combination of bought, packaged food known as "fueling." These mini-meals that the company sells are designed to fill you full and help you lose weight to lean and green recipes(homemade). There's no carbohydrates or calories counting. Usually, as part of six-or-so mini-meals every day, members add water to dried food or unwrap a snack. Furthermore, the method advises performing around 30 minutes of a normal, moderately intense workout. The Optavia diet is a regimen that offers three food programs from which you can choose: Optimal Weight 5 & 1 Method, Optimal Weight 4 & 2 & 1 Method, and Optimal Health 3 & 3 Program. The latter is oriented toward maintaining weight. Each schedule recommends consuming a certain amount of "Fuelings," which are prepackaged by Optavia brand snacks or meals. These diets provide more than the government's guideline that 10- 35 % of the total calories come from protein. Optavia's half of the diet plan or even more of its "fuelings," including cereal, bars, cookies, shakes, and few savory choices, like smashed potatoes, soup. These packaged foods have whey protein, soy protein as the first ingredient.

Lean & green meals compromise the rest of the diet, which you prepare on your own by your store-bought ingredients. Those include:

- Three portions of vegetables(non-starchy) like cucumbers, greens, lettuce, and celery
- 5 to 7 (cooked)ounces of lean protein like egg whites, fish, soy, chicken, and turkey
- 2 portions of healthy fats like avocado oil, olive oil, and olives

How Optavia Diet Works

There are three different low-calorie options to select from based on your personal goal. Five Optaviafuelings and one lean & green meal consisting of vegetables and proteins like chicken and broccoli are part of the 5&1 Menu. The 4&2&1 strategy requires four fuelings, two lean & green meals, and one light snack that could be like a fruit slice. The organization provides the 3&3 option for weight management, which involves three fuelings and the same amount of three lean & green meals. Dieters are assisted by their Optavia mentor and

an online dieter group with guidance and inspiration.

They have advertised items named OptaviaFuelings, and organic entrées known as Lean & Green meals, but you can pick from many choices.

OptaviaFuelings

OptaviaFuelings contains over 60 products that are low in carbohydrates but rich in protein and probiotic cultures that have helpful bacteria that will improve your stomach's health. These items contain puddings, bars, cookies, pasta, shakes, cereals, and soups.

While they can seem to be very high in carbohydrates, they are built to be lower in sugar and carbohydrates than conventional variants of the same foods. optavia replaces sugar and limited serving sizes to do this.

In comparison, several fuels are packaged with soy protein isolate and whey protein powder.

Diet Plans

- **5&1 Plan.** This is the most popular Plan, this Plan includes five Optavia-Fuelings and one Lean & Green meal each day. This Plan is made for **rapid weight loss.**
- **4&2&1 Plan.** This Plan is designed for those who
- require more flexibility or calories in diet plan choices. This Plan includes 4 OptaviaFuelings, 2 Lean & Green meals, and one **snack** each day.
- **3&3 Plan.** This Plan is designed to maintain weight; this one includes 3 OptaviaFuelings and 3 balanced Lean & Green meals per day.

Optavia's 3&3 and 4&2&1 plan combine real meals with meal substitutes. People who want to lose weight gradually or maintain current weight, these plans are best-suited for those. All these lean & green meals and fuelings are best kept in a specific calorie range according to your Plan.

How to Follow the Optavia Diet?

To follow the diet first off, you must start with a conversation with the Optavia diet coach to determine which Optavia plan is best suited for your goal. It could be weight loss or weight maintenance, and make yourself familiar with the Plan.

Initial Steps

Most people begin with the Optimum Weight 5&1 Diet for weight reduction, an 800 to 1,000 calorie routine that will help you lose 12 pounds over12 weeks. You are expected to consume one meal every 2,3 hours and have moderate activity for half an hour on some days of the week. In general, no more than 100 grams of carbs are given per day by the Fuelings and portions. As Optavia coaches get paid on commission, you will order these meals from your coach's specific page.

Lean and Green meals aim to be high in protein and low in carbs. One meal provides 5, 7(cooked) ounces of lean protein, 3 portions of vegetables mostly non-starchy, and up to 2 portions of good fats. This schedule also involves one extra snack a day, which the coach would accept. 3 celery sticks, half a cup of sugar-free gelatin, or a half-ounce of nuts are Plan-approved treats. Bear in mind that the 5&1 Strategy does not allow alcohol to consume.

Maintenance Phase

When you achieve the target weight, you begin a six-week maintenance period,

which entails steadily raising calories to 1,550 calories but not more than that each day and incorporating low-fat dairy, whole grains, and fruits in a larger range of foods.

You are expected to switch over to the Ideal Wellness 3&3 Schedule after six weeks, which involves 3 Lean & Green meals and 3 Fuels every day, with regular Optavia coaching. Many who have had continuous progress on the platform have the possibility of being qualified as a coach for Optavia.

Optavia Diet's Essentials

Food is further divided for your convenience.

Compliant Foods

- Greens and other non-starchy vegetables
- Optaviafuelings
- Lean meats
- Low-fat dairy and whole grains
- Healthy fats
- Fresh fruit

Non-Compliant Foods

- Sugary beverages
- High-calorie additions
- Alcohol
- Indulgent desserts

Lean Meats

- For lean & green, you require to consume 5,7 ounces of lean meat.
- **Lean meat is** lamb, **salmon** & **pork chops**
- **Leaner meat is chicken breast** or swordfish
- **The leanest meat is egg whites,** cod, and shrimp

Greens Portions

- 5 & 1 Optavia program asks you to consume two **non-starchy vegetable** portions, alongside the protein in your lean & green meal.
- **Lower carb is Salad greens**
- **Moderate carb are summer squash** or **cauliflower**
- **Higher carbs are** peppers and Broccoli

Food List for the Optavia Diet's Fueling

- Turkey meatball marinara

- Snack or meal-replacement bars
- Smoothies
- Beef stew
- Shakes
- **Chicken** with **rice** & vegetables
- Popcorn
- Smashed potatoes
- Chicken cacciatore
- Wild rice & chicken soup
- Cereal
- Pancakes
- Rustic tomato herb penne
- Cookies
- Mac & cheese

Foods suggested for making Lean & Green meals include

- Fish: swordfish, cod, **tilapia**, flounder, and tuna
- Shellfish: scallops, crab, and shrimp
- Buffalo meat
- Ground meat at least 85 % leaner
- **Egg** whites
- Healthy fat like canola oil, **olive oil**, olives, **avocado**, and low-carb salad dressing
- Lean beef
- Whole eggs only three each week
- Turkey or Chicken
- **Tofu**
- Tenderloin or Pork chop
- Vegetables like cucumbers, leafy greens, **asparagus**, radishes, mushrooms, and **broccoli**

Chapter 1: Optavia Lean & Green Poultry Air-Fry Recipes

1.1 Teriyaki Chicken Drumsticks with Salad Greens

(Prep Time: 30 mints | Cook Time:20 mints | Servings: 6)

Ingredients

- Six chicken drumsticks
- Teriyaki sauce: one cup
- Salad greens: one cup
- Sesame seeds and chopped green onion, for garnish

Instructions

- Let the air-fryer preheat to 360F.
- Pour teriyaki sauce in a big zip lock bag, add in chicken drumsticks.
- Mix them so well coated. Let it marinate for half an hour.
- Put drumsticks in a single layer in the air fryer basket, let it cook for 20 minutes.
- Shake the basket multiple times for even cooking.
- Top with green onions, sesame seeds, and serve with the side of salad greens.

Nutritional value: per serving: Calories: 163kcal | Carbohydrates: 7g | Protein: 16g | Fat: 7g |

1.2 Air Fried Philly Cheesesteak Taquitos

(Prep Time: 20 mints | Cook Time: 6-8 hours | Servings: 6)

Ingredients

- Dry Italian dressing mix: one package
- Super Soft Corn Tortillas: one pack
- Green peppers: two pieces, chopped
- One white onion, diced
- 12 cups of lean beef steak strips
- Beef stock: 2 cups
- Lettuce shredded, one cup
- Provolone cheese: ten slices
- Olive oil

Instructions

- In a slow cooker, add onion, beef, stock, bell pepper, and seasonings.
- Cover it and let it cook on low 6 or 8 hours.
- Heat tortillas for two minutes in the microwave.
- Let the air fryer preheated at 350F.
- Take cheesesteak out from slow cooker, spoon 2-3 tablespoon of steak in the tortilla.
- Add some of the cheese, roll tortilla tightly, and put in an air fryer basket.
- Prepare as many tortillas as you want.
- Brush lightly with olive oil
- Cook for 6-8 minutes.
- Flip the tortillas and brush more oil if required.

- Serve with shredded lettuce and enjoy

Nutritional value: per serving: calories 210| carbs 20g| protein 23 |fat 14g

1.3 Air Fryer Nashville Hot Chicken with Spinach Salad

(Prep Time: 30 mints| Cook Time:25 mints| Servings: 8)

Ingredients

- Buttermilk: 2 cups
- Chicken thighs(bone-in): 8
- Cayenne pepper: 1 tsp.
- Hot sauce: 1/4 cup
- Garlic powder: 2 Tbsp.
- Salt: 1 tsp.
- Low-fat butter: 1/2 cup
- Flour: 2 cups
- Black pepper: 1 tsp.
- Old bay: 1 tsp.
- Paprika: 1 tsp.

Instructions

- In a mixing bowl, add hot sauce and buttermilk, mix it well, then add chicken pieces.
- Marinate in the refrigerator for 1 to 24 hours.
- In a bowl, add garlic powder, flour, salt, black pepper, paprika, cayenne pepper, and old bay. Mix well.
- Always cook the chicken in a single layer, in the air fryer
- Take chicken out from buttermilk, coat in the flour mix. Let the chicken rest on a cooling rack for 15 minutes before putting in the air fryer.
- Place the breaded chicken in the air fryer, leaving room between the pieces.
- Cook for 25 minutes, at 390 F. after halftime, take the basket out and spray the chicken with olive oil
- This step is optional. Mix two tbsp. Of hot sauce with melted butter. Brush the cooked crispy chicken with it.
- Serve with the spinach salad.

Nutritional value: per serving: calories 330|Fat 20g|Carbs 19g|protein 26g

1.4 Air Fryer Italian Sausage & Vegetables

(Prep Time: 5 mints| Cook Time:14 mints| Servings: 4)

Ingredients

- One bell pepper
- Italian Sausage: 4 pieces spicy or sweet
- One small onion
- 1/4 cup of mushrooms

Instructions

- Let the air fryer pre-heat to 400 F for three minutes.
- Put Italian sausage in a single layer in the air fryer basket and let it cook for six minutes.
- Slice the vegetables while the sausages are cooking.

- After six minutes, reduce the temperature to 360 F. flip the sausage halfway through. Add the mushrooms, onions, and peppers in the basket around the sausage.
- Cook at 360 F for 8 minutes. After a 4-minute mix around the sausage and vegetables.
- With an instant-read thermometer, the sausage temperature should be 160 F.
- Cook more for few minutes if the temperature is not 160F.
- Take vegetables and sausage out and serve hot with brown rice.

Nutritional value: per serving: calories 291 | fat: 21g | carbs 10g | Protein: 16g

1.5 Air Fryer Dumplings

(Prep Time: 5 mints | Cook Time:10 mints | Servings: 3)

Ingredients

- One packet of frozen chicken, vegetable, or pork dumplings
- Salad greens: one cup
- Dipping sauce
- Maple syrup: 1/8 cup
- Soy sauce: 1/4 cup
- Red pepper flakes: Pinch
- Garlic powder: 1/2 tsp.
- Rice vinegar: 1/2 tsp.
- Water: 1/4 cup

Instructions

- Let the air fryer pre-heat to 370 degrees for four minutes.
- Put the dumplings in the air fryer basket in a single layer and spray with oil.
- Let it air fry for five minutes, toss the basket, spray with a little more oil.
- Let them cook for another six minutes.
- In the meantime, add all dipping sauce ingredients in a bowl and mix well.
- Take the dumpling out and serve with salad greens.

Nutritional value: per serving: Cal 233 | FAT: 7g | Carbs: 26g | Protein: 18g

1.6 Air Fryer Chicken Wings with Buffalo Sauce

(Prep Time: 5 mints | Cook Time:25 mints | Servings: 6)

Ingredients

- Chicken drumettes & flats: 4 cups
- Salt & pepper, to taste

Buffalo Sauce

- Hot sauce: 1/2 cup
- White vinegar: 2 tablespoons
- Melted butter: 1/2 cup
- Worcestershire sauce: 2 teaspoons
- Pinch of garlic powder

Instructions

- Let the air fryer preheat to 380F.

- Separate the wings, making a flat and drumsticks, discarding the tips.
- With paper towels, pat dry the chicken wings, sprinkle generously salt and pepper, and other seasonings of your choice.
- Put them in an air-fryer basket and cook for about 22 minutes.
- After that increase, the temperature to 400 degrees, cook for more five minutes for chicken skin to get crispy.
- Mix all ingredients of buffalo sauce and mix well.
- Coat the wings with homemade buffalo sauce.
- Serve with the side of salad greens.

Nutritional value: per serving: Cal 315| Fat: 20g| Carbs: 1g|Protein: 30g

1.7 Air Fryer Grilled Chicken Recipe

(Prep Time: 30 mints| Cook Time:20 mints| Servings: 3)

Ingredients

- Chicken tenders: 4 cups

Marinade

- Honey: 2 Tbsp.
- Olive oil: 1/4 cup
- White vinegar: 2 Tbsp.
- Water: 2 Tbsp.
- Half teaspoon salt
- Garlic powder: 1 tsp.
- Half teaspoon of paprika
- Onion powder: 1 tsp.
- Half teaspoon crushed red pepper

Instructions

- In a mixing bowl, add all ingredients of the marinade and mix well.
- Then add the chicken mix to coat. Cover with plastic wrap, and marinate in the refrigerator for half an hour.
- Put chicken tenders in the air fryer basket in one even layer.
- Cook for 3 minutes at 390 F. flip the tenders over and cook for five minutes more or until chicken is completely cooked through.
- Serve with the side of salad greens.

Nutritional value: per serving: calories 230|fat 14g| protein 20 g| carbs 11g

1.8 Air-Fried Chicken Pie

(Prep Time: 10 mints| Cook Time: 30 mints| Servings: 2)

Ingredients

- Puff pastry: 2 sheets
- Chicken thighs: 2 pieces, cut into cubes
- One small onion, chopped
- Small potatoes: 2, chopped
- Mushrooms: 1/4 cup
- Light soya sauce
- One carrot, chopped
- Black pepper, to taste
- Worcestershire sauce: to taste
- Salt, to taste
- Italian mixed dried herbs

- Garlic powder: a pinch
- Plain flour: 2 tbsp.
- Milk, as required
- Melted butter

Instructions

- In a mixing bowl, add light soya sauce and pepper add the chicken cubes and coat well.
- In a pan over medium heat, sauté carrot, potatoes, and onion. Add some water, if required, to cook the vegetables.
- Add the chicken cubes and mushrooms and cook them too.
- Stir in black pepper, salt, Worcestershire sauce, garlic powder, and dried herbs.
- When the chicken is cooked through, add some of the flour and mix well.
- Add in the milk and let the vegetables simmer until tender.
- Place one piece of puff pastry in the baking tray of air fryer, poke holes with a fork.
- Add on top the cooked chicken filling and eggs and puff pastry on top, with
- holes. Cut the excess pastry off. Glaze with oil spray or melted butter
- Air fry at 180 F, for six mints or until it becomes golden brown.
- Serve with microgreens.

Nutritional value: per serving: calories 224|protein 20g|fat 18 g| carbs 17g

1.9 Air-Fried Buttermilk Chicken

(Prep Time: 30 mints| Cook Time:20 mints| Servings: 6)

Ingredients

- Chicken thighs: 4 cups skin-on, bone-in

Marinade

- Buttermilk: 2 cups
- Black pepper: 2 tsp.
- Cayenne pepper: 1 tsp.
- Salt: 2 tsp.

Seasoned Flour

- Baking powder: 1 tbsp.
- All-purpose flour: 2 cups
- Paprika powder: 1 tbsp.
- Salt: 1 tsp.
- Garlic powder: 1 tbsp.

Instructions

- Let the air fry heat at 180 C.
- With a paper towel, pat dry the chicken thighs.
- In a mixing bowl, add paprika, black pepper, salt mix well, then add chicken pieces. Add buttermilk and coat the chicken well. Let it marinate for at least 6 hours.
- In another bowl, add baking powder, salt, flour, pepper, and paprika. Put one by one of the chicken pieces and coat in the seasoning mix.
- Spray oil on chicken pieces and place breaded chicken skin side up in air fryer basket in one layer, cook for 8 minutes, then flip the chicken pieces' cook for another ten minutes

- Take out and serve with salad greens.

Nutritional value: per serving: Cal 210|fat 18 g| protein 22g|carbs 12 g

1.10 Low Carb Parmesan Chicken Meatballs

(Prep Time: 10 mints| Cook Time:12 mints| Servings: 20)

Ingredients

- Pork rinds: half cup, ground
- Ground chicken: 4 cups
- Parmesan cheese: half cup grated
- Kosher salt: 1 tsp.
- Garlic powder: 1 tsp.
- One egg beaten
- Paprika: 1 tsp.
- Pepper: half tsp.

Breading

- Pork rinds: half cup ground

Instructions

- Let the Air Fryer pre-heat to 400°F.
- Add cheese, chicken, egg, pepper, half cup of pork rinds, garlic, salt, and paprika in a big mixing ball. Mix well into a dough, make into 1and half-inch balls.
- Coat the meatballs in pork rinds(ground).
- Oil sprays the air fry basket and add meatballs in one even layer.
- Let it cook for 12 minutes at 400°F, flipping once halfway through.
- Serve with salad greens.

Nutritional value: per serving: Cal 240| fat 10 g| carbs 12.1 g| protein 19.9 g

1.11 Sriracha-Honey Chicken Wings

(Prep Time: 30 mints| Cook Time:15 mints| Servings: 2)

Ingredients

- Soy sauce: 1 and 1/2 tablespoons
- Chicken wings: 4 cups
- Sriracha sauce: 2 tablespoons
- Butter: 1 tablespoon
- Half cup honey
- Juice of half lime
- Scallion's cilantro, and chives for garnish

Instructions

- Let the air fryer pre-heat to 360 degrees F.
- Put the chicken wings to an air fryer basket, cook for half an hour, flip the wings every seven minutes, and cook thoroughly.
- Meanwhile, in a saucepan, add all the ingredients of the sauce and simmer for three minutes.
- Take out the chicken wings and coat them in sauce well.
- Garnish with scallions. Serve with a microgreen salad.

Nutritional value: per serving: Calories 207 |Proteins 22g |Carbs 10g|Fat 15g |

1.12 Air Fryer Chicken Cheese Quesadilla

(Prep Time: 4 mints| Cook Time: 7 mints| Servings: 4)

Ingredients

- Precooked chicken: one cup, diced
- Tortillas: 2 pieces
- Low-fat cheese: one cup (shredded)

Instructions

- Spray oil the air basket and place one tortilla in it. Add cooked chicken and cheese on top.
- Add the second tortilla on top. Put a metal rack on top.
- Cook for 6 minutes at 370 degrees, flip it halfway through so cooking evenly.
- Slice and serve with salad greens

Nutritional value: per serving: Calories: 171kcal | Carbohydrates: 8g | Protein: 15g | Fat: 8g |

1.13 Air Fried Empanadas

(Prep Time: 10 mints| Cook Time:20 mints| Servings: 2)

Ingredients

- Square gyoza wrappers: eight pieces
- Olive oil: 1 tablespoon
- White onion: 1/4 cup, finely diced
- Mushrooms: 1/4 cup, finely diced
- Half cup lean ground beef
- Chopped garlic: 2 teaspoons
- Paprika: 1/4 teaspoon
- Ground cumin: 1/4 teaspoon
- Six green olives, diced
- Ground cinnamon: 1/8 teaspoon
- Diced tomatoes: half cup
- One egg, lightly beaten

Instructions

- In a skillet, over a medium flame, add oil, onions, and beef and cook for 3 minutes, until beef turns brown.
- Add mushrooms, and cook for six minutes until it starts to brown. Then add paprika, cinnamon, olives, cumin, and garlic and cook for 3 minutes or more.
- Add in the chopped tomatoes, and cook for a minute. Turn off the heat; let it cool for five minutes.
- Lay gyoza wrappers on a flat surface add one and a half tbsp. of beef filling in each wrapper. Brush edges with water or egg, fold wrappers, pinch edges.
- Put four empanadas in even layer in an air fryer basket, and cook for 7 minutes at 400°F until nicely browned.
- Serve with sauce and salad greens.

Nutritional value: per serving Calories 343 |Fat 19g |Protein 18g |Carbohydrate 12.9g

1.14 Air Fryer BBQ Chicken Wings

(Prep Time: 5 mints| Cook Time: 15 mints| Servings: 4)

Ingredients

- BBQ sauce: half cup
- Chicken wings: 4 cups
- Black pepper, to taste

- Garlic powder: 1/8 teaspoon
- Ranch
- Celery sticks

Instructions

- Let Air Fryer preheat to 400 degrees.
- With paper towels, pat dry the chicken wings, rub the garlic powder on them. Put them in the air fryer, in one even layer.
- Let it cook for 15 minutes, flip the wings once or twice. Cook for another 3 minutes for crispy skin.
- Take them out from the air fryer and toss them in BBQ sauce. toss well to coat
- Serve with celery sticks, mixed greens, and ranch dressing.

Nutritional value: per serving: Calories: 197kcal | Carbohydrates: 14g | Protein: 11g | Fat: 10g

1.15 Air Fryer Cornish Hen

(Prep Time: 5 mints| Cook Time:25 mints| Servings: 3)

Ingredients

- One Cornish hen
- Salt & black pepper, to taste
- Olive oil spray
- Paprika, ¼ tbsp.

Instructions

- Mix all spices and Rub the spices all over Cornish hen.
- Spray the air fryer basket with olive oil.
- Put Cornish hen in an Air fryer.
- Cook for 25 minutes at 390 F. flip after half time.
- Serve with a mixed green salad.

Nutritional value: per serving: Calories: 300 | Protein: 25g | Fat: 21g | carbs: 20 g

1.16 Air Fry Rib-Eye Steak

(Prep Time: 5 mints| Cook Time: 14 mints| Servings: 2)

Ingredients

- Lean rib eye steaks: 2, medium size
- Salt & freshly ground black pepper, to taste

Instructions

- Let the air fry preheat at 400 F. pat dry steaks with paper towels.
- Use any spice blend or just salt and pepper on steaks.
- Generously on both sides of the steak.
- Put steaks in the air fryer basket. Cook according to the rareness you want.

  Or cook for 14 minutes and flip after half time.
- Take out from the air fryer and let it rest for about 5 minutes.
- Serve with micro green salad.

Nutritional value: per serving: Calories: 470kcal | Protein: 45g | Fat: 31g | carbs: 23 g

1.17 Orange Chicken Wings

(Prep Time: 5 mints| Cook Time: 14 mints| Servings: 2)

Ingredients

- Honey: 1 tbsp.
- Chicken Wings, Six pieces
- One orange zest and juice
- Worcestershire Sauce: 1.5 tbsp.
- Black pepper, to taste
- Herbs (sage, rosemary, oregano, parsley, basil, thyme, and mint)

Instructions

- Wash and pat dry the chicken wings
- In a bowl, add chicken wings, pour zest and orange juice
- Add the rest of the ingredients and rub on chicken wings. Let it marinate for at least half an hour.
- Let the Air fryer preheat at 180°C
- In an aluminum foil, wrap the marinated wings and put them in an air fryer and cook for 20 minutes at 180 C
- After 20 minutes, remove aluminum foil and brush the sauce over wings and cook for 15 minutes more. Then again, brush the sauce and cook for another ten minutes.
- Take out from the air fryer and serve with salad greens.

Nutritional value: per serving: Calories 271 |Proteins 29g |Carbs 20g |Fat

15g |

1.18 Lemon Rosemary Chicken

(Prep Time: 30 mints| Cook Time:20 mints| Servings: 2)

Ingredients

For marinade

- Chicken: 2 and ½ cups
- Ginger: 1 tsp, minced
- Olive oil: 1/2 tbsp.
- Soy sauce: 1 tbsp.

For the sauce

- Half lemon
- Honey: 3 tbsp.
- Oyster sauce: 1 tbsp.
- Fresh rosemary: half cup, chopped

Instructions

- In a big mixing bowl, add the marinade ingredients with chicken, and mix well.
- Keep in the refrigerator for at least half an hour.
- Let the oven preheat to 200 C for three minutes.
- Place the marinated chicken in the air fryer in a single layer. And cook for 6 minutes at 200 degrees.
- Meanwhile, add all the sauces ingredients in a bowl and mix well except for lemon wedges.
- Brush the sauce generously over half-baked chicken add lemon juice on top.
- Cook for another 13 min at 200 C. flip the chicken halfway through. Let the chicken evenly brown.

- Serve with micro greens salad.

Nutrition Value: per serving: Calories 308 |Proteins 25g |Carbs 7g|Fat 12 g |

1.19 Crumbed Chicken Tenderloins

(Prep Time: 10 mints| Cook Time:12 mints| Servings: 4)

Ingredients

- Eight chicken tenderloins
- Olive oil: 2 tablespoons
- One egg whisked
- 1/4 cup breadcrumbs

Instructions

- Let the air fryer heat to 180 C.
- In a big bowl, add breadcrumbs and oil, mix well until forms a crumbly mixture
- Dip chicken tenderloin in whisked egg and coat in breadcrumbs mixture.
- Place the breaded chicken in the air fryer and cook at 180C for 12 minutes or more.
- Take out from the air fryer and serve with the side of salad greens.

Nutritional value: per serving: Calories 206|Proteins 20g |Carbs 17g |Fat 10g |

1.20 Beef Schnitzel (Air Fried)

(Prep Time: 10 mints| Cook Time:15 mints| Servings: 1)

Ingredients

- One lean beef schnitzel
- Olive oil: 2 tablespoon
- Breadcrumbs: ¼ cup
- One egg
- One lemon, to serve

Instructions

- Let the air fryer heat to 180 C.
- In a big bowl, add breadcrumbs and oil, mix well until forms a crumbly mixture
- Dip beef steak in whisked egg and coat in breadcrumbs mixture.
- Place the breaded beef in the air fryer and cook at 180C for 15 minutes or more until fully cooked through.
- Take out from the air fryer and serve with the side of salad greens and lemon.

Nutrition Value: per serving: Calories 340 |Proteins 20g |Carbs 14g |Fat 10g

|Fiber 7g

1.21 Air Fried Tom Yum Chicken Wings

(Prep Time: 30 mints| Cook Time:20 mints| Servings: 3)

Ingredients

- Tom Yum Paste: 2 tbsp.
- 8 Chicken Wings
- Water: 1 tbsp.

COATING

- Corn flour: 2 tbsp.
- Baking Powder: half teaspoon
- Tapioca Starch: 2 tbsp.

Instructions

- Mix Tom Yum paste with water in a small bowl.
- Add chicken wings in the tom yum mixture, coat well, and keep marinade in the refrigerator for four hours.
- Let the Air fryer preheat at 180°C.
- In a mixing bowl, mix tapioca starch, baking powder, and corn flour and mix well. Coat the chicken in the flour mix. Spray the oil on chicken.
- Place the chicken in the air fryer in even layer and cook for 10-12 minutes
- Flip them once and cook for more 5,8 mines
- Take them out from the air fryer and serve with salad greens and lemon wedges

Nutritional value: per serving: Calories 320 |Proteins 27g |Carbs 18g|Fat 14g |Fiber 5g

1.22 Air Fryer Ravioli

(Prep Time: 10 mints| Cook Time:10 mints| Servings: 6)

Ingredients

- Olive oil: 1 teaspoon
- Italian-style bread crumbs: 2 cups
- Homemade marinara sauce
- Cheese ravioli with cooked chicken: 12 pieces
- Parmesan cheese: 1/4 cup
- Buttermilk: 1 cup

Instructions

- Add cheese and chicken to dumpling wrappers, and with water seal the edges.
- Then coat ravioli in buttermilk.
- In a mixing bowl, add olive oil and breadcrumbs, mix them well, and add ravioli to the mixture
- Place breaded ravioli in the air fryer basket on baking paper.
- Let it cook for five minutes at 200°F
- Serve with salad greens and marinara sauce for dipping.

Nutritional Value: per serving: Calories 218 |Proteins 14g |Carbs 11g |Fat 18g

1.23 Air Fried Spicy Chicken Wings

(Prep Time: 30 mints| Cook Time:20 mints| Servings: 2)

Ingredients

- Honey: 1 tbsp.
- Chicken Wings: 6 pcs
- Cloves of minced Garlic
- Worcestershire Sauce: 2 tbsp.
- Chili Flakes: 1 tsp.
- Salt & pepper, to taste
- Cooking Spray

Instructions

- Wash and pat dry the chicken wings.
- In a bowl, mix chili flakes, salt, Worcestershire sauce, pepper, and honey. Mix well and add the chicken wings to it and let it marinate for at least an hour.

- Drizzle olive oil on marinated chicken wings
- Place the chicken wings in the air fryer basket, and cook for 8 minutes at 160 C.
- Flip halfway and cook for more than four minutes.
- Serve with air-fried zucchini.

Nutritional value: per serving: Calories 300 |Proteins 28g |Carbs 11 g |Fat 18g |

1.24 Air Fryer Chicken & Broccoli

(Prep Time: 10 mints| Cook Time:15 mints| Servings: 4)

Ingredients

- Olive oil: 2 Tablespoons
- Chicken breast: 4 cups, bone and skinless (cut into cubes)
- Half medium onion, roughly sliced
- Low sodium soy sauce: 1 Tbsp.
- Garlic powder: half teaspoon
- Rice vinegar: 2 teaspoons
- Broccoli: 1-2 cups, cut into florets
- Hot sauce: 2 teaspoons
- Fresh minced ginger: 1 Tbsp.
- Sesame seed oil: 1 teaspoon
- Salt & black pepper, to taste

Instructions

- In a bowl, add chicken breast, onion, and broccoli. Combine them well.
- In another bowl, add ginger, oil, sesame oil, rice vinegar, hot sauce, garlic powder, and soy sauce mix it well. Then add the broccoli, chicken, and onions to marinade.
- Coat well the chicken with sauces. And let it rest in the refrigerator for 15 minutes
- Place chicken mix in one even layer in air fryer basket and cook for 16-20 minutes, at 380 F. halfway through, toss the basket gently and cook the chicken evenly
- Add five minutes more, if required.
- Add salt and pepper, if needed.
- serve warm with lemon wedges

Nutritional value: per serving:
Calories 191 |**Fat** 7g|**Carbohydrates** 4g|**P rotein** 25g

1.25 Air Fried Maple Chicken Thighs

(Prep Time: 10 mints| Cook Time:25mints| Servings: 4)

Ingredient

- One egg
- Buttermilk: 1 cup
- Maple syrup: half cup
- Chicken thighs: 4 pieces
- Granulated garlic: 1 tsp.

Dry Mix

- Granulated garlic: half tsp.
- All-purpose flour: half cup
- Salt: one tbsp.
- Sweet paprika: one tsp.
- Smoked paprika: half tsp.
- Tapioca flour: ¼ cup

- Cayenne pepper: ¼ teaspoon
- Granulated onion: one tsp.
- Black pepper: ¼ teaspoon
- Honey powder: half tsp.

Instructions

- In a zip lock bag, add egg, one tsp. of granulated garlic, buttermilk, and maple syrup, add in the chicken thighs and let it marinate for one hour or more in the refrigerator
- In a mixing bowl, add sweet paprika, tapioca flour, granulated onion, half tsp. of granulated garlic, flour, cayenne pepper, salt, pepper, honey powder, and smoked paprika mix it well.
- Let the air fry preheat to 380 F
- Coat the marinated chicken thighs in the dry spice mix, shake the excess off.
- Put the chicken skin side down in the air fryer
- Let it cook for 12 minutes. Flip thighs halfway through and cook for 13 minutes more.
- Serve with salad greens.

Nutritional value: per serving: 415.4 calories| protein 23.3g| carbohydrates 20.8g| fat 13.4g

1.26 General Tso's Chicken

(Prep Time: 5 mints| Cook Time:25 mints| Servings: 4)

Ingredients

- Chicken thighs: 8 cups boneless, skinless (cubed)
- 3 green onions, roughly chopped
- **Corn starch:** 2 tsp
- Vegetable oil: 1 Tbsp.
- Rice vinegar: 2 Tbsp.
- Six red chilies, dried
- Potato starch: 1/3 cup
- Garlic minced: 2 tsp
- Brown sugar: 3/4 cup
- Chicken broth: half cup
- Ginger minced: 1 tsp
- Soy sauce: half cup
- Sesame oil: 1 tsp
- Salt, to taste
- Cup water: 1/4

Instructions

- Let the air fryer preheat to 400 F.
- In a bowl, add potato starch and chicken thighs, coat them well. Add chicken thigs to the air fryer in one even layer and cooks for 25 minutes.
- Shake the air fryer basket after every 5-7 minutes.
- In the meantime, heat olive oil in a pan over medium heat and add garlic, ginger, dried chilies, and green onions, cook for one minute, until onions have softened.
- Stir in soy sauce, sesame oil, chicken broth, a pinch of salt, brown sugar, rice vinegar, and mix well. Let it boil and cook for three minutes.
- Then add air fried chicken in sauce and coat well.
- Stir in the corn starch mix (with water), cook for one minute.

- Serve with boiled vegetables and enjoy.

Nutritional value: per serving: Calories: 430|fat 20 g| protein 23 g| carbs 20.1 g|

1.27 Crispy Korean Air Fried Chicken Wings

(Prep Time: 10 mints| Cook Time: 30 mints| Servings: 4)

Ingredients

- Chicken wings: 4 cups
- Onion powder: 1 tsp
- Corn starch: ¾ cup
- Garlic powder: 1 tsp
- Salt: ½ tsp

Korean Air Fried Chicken Sauce

- **Soy sauce:** 1 Tbsp.
- Korean chili paste: 2 Tbsp.
- **Honey:** 3 Tbsp.
- Ginger minced: 1 tsp
- Garlic minced: 1 tsp
- **Brown sugar:** 2 Tbsp.
- Half tsp. salt

Instructions

- Wash and pat dry the chicken wings, in a bowl, add ½ tsp of salt, onion powder,
- and garlic powder then add chicken wings and coat them well
- Then coat the wings in corn starch. And put them in the air fryer.
- Let the wings cook at 390 F for half an hour. Rotate every ten minutes.

Korean Sauce

- In a saucepan, over medium flame, add all ingredients and let it boil and simmer for five minutes. Turn the heat off
- Add cooked wings to the sauce and coat well.
- Serve with steamed vegetables.

Nutritional value: per serving: Calories: 340 | Carbohydrates: 24g | Protein: 23g | Fat: 19g |

1.28 Air Fryer Meatloaf

(Prep Time: 10 mints| Cook Time:40 mints| Servings: 8)

Ingredients

- Ground lean beef: 4 cups
- Bread crumbs: 1 cup (soft and fresh)
- Chopped mushrooms: ½ cup
- Cloves of minced garlic
- Shredded carrots: ½ cup
- Beef broth: ¼ cup
- Chopped onions: ½ cup
- Two eggs beaten
- Ketchup: 3 Tbsp.
- Worcestershire sauce: 1 Tbsp.
- Dijon mustard: 1 Tbsp.

For Glaze

- Honey: ¼ cup
- Ketchup: half cup

- Dijon mustard: 2 tsp

Instructions

- In a big bowl, add beef broth and breadcrumbs, stir well. And set it aside in a food processor, add garlic, onions, mushrooms, and carrots and pulse on high until finely chopped
- In a separate bowl, add soaked breadcrumbs, Dijon mustard, Worcestershire
- sauce, eggs, lean ground beef, ketchup, and salt. With your hands, combine well and make it into a loaf.
- Let the air fryer preheat to 390 F.
- Put Meatloaf in the Air Fryer and let it cook for 45 minutes.
- In the meantime, add Dijon mustard, ketchup, and brown sugar in a bowl and mix. Glaze this mix over Meatloaf when five minutes are left.
- Rest the Meatloaf after for ten minutes before serving.

Nutritional value: per serving: Calories 330 | Proteins 19g | Carbs 16g | Fat 9.9 g |

1.29 Air Fryer Spicy Chicken & Vegetables

(Prep Time: 20 mints | Cook Time:30 mints | Servings: 2)

Ingredients

Spiced Chicken

- Chicken breasts: 2 skinless, boneless
- Onion powder: half tsp.
- Olive oil: 1/2 Tbsp.
- Chili powder: 1 tsp.
- Cumin: 1/4 tsp.
- Paprika: half tsp.
- Salt: half tsp.
- Garlic powder: half tsp.
- Pepper: half tsp.

Vegetables

- Carrots: 2-3 large
- Onion: one red
- Olive oil: 1/2 Tbsp.
- Chopped scallions
- Pinch of salt

Instructions

- Let the air fryer preheat to 325 F
- In a big bowl, add all chicken spices and make a spice mix. Then add chicken breasts with half tbsp. of olive oil and coat well. Set it aside.
- Cut the vegetables according to your preference. Cut onions in layers, and separate each layer, coat all the vegetables with half tbsp. of olive oil and salt
- Lay vegetables in the air fryer first, then add chicken on top—Cook for almost 35 minutes or more. Flip the chicken halfway through, and toss the vegetables.
- Serve hot.

Nutritional value: per serving: Calories: 344cal | Carbohydrates: 34g | Protein: 28g | Fat: 11g |

1.30 Air Fried Steak with Asparagus Bundles

(Prep Time: 20 mints| Cook Time:30 mints| Servings: 2)

Ingredients

- Olive oil spray
- Flank steak (2 pounds)- cut into 6 pieces
- Kosher salt and black pepper
- Two cloves of minced garlic
- Asparagus: 4 cups
- Tamari sauce: half cup
- Three bell peppers: sliced thinly
- Beef broth: 1/3 cup
- 1 Tbsp. of unsalted butter
- Balsamic vinegar: 1/4 cup

Instructions

- Sprinkle salt and pepper on steak, and rub.
- In a zip lock bag, add garlic and Tamari sauce, then add steak, toss well and seal the bag.
- Let it marinate for one hour to overnight.
- Equally, place bell peppers and asparagus in the center of the steak.
- Roll the steak around the vegetables and secure well with toothpicks.
- Preheat the air fryer.
- Spray the steak with olive oil spray. And place steaks in the air fryer.
- Cook for 15 minutes at 400 degrees or more till steaks are cooked
- Take the steak out from the air fryer and let it rest for five minute
- Remove steak bundles and allow them to rest for 5 minutes before serving/slicing.
- In the meantime, add butter, balsamic vinegar, and broth over medium flame. Mix well and reduce it by half. Add salt and pepper to taste.
- Pour over steaks right before serving.

Nutritional value: per serving: Calories 471 |Proteins 29g |Carbs 20g |Fat 15g |

1.31 Air Fryer Beef Steak Kabobs with Vegetables

(Prep Time: 30 mints| Cook Time:10 mints| Servings: 4)

Ingredients

- Soy sauce: 2 tbsp.
- Lean beef chuck ribs: 4 cups, cut into one-inch pieces
- Low-fat sour cream: 1/3 cup
- Half onion
- 8 skewers: 6 inch
- One bell peppers

Instructions

- In a mixing bowl, add soy sauce and sour cream, mix well. Add the lean beef chunks, coat well, and let it marinate for half an hour or more.
- Cut onion, bell pepper in one-inch pieces. In water, soak skewers for ten minutes.

- Add onions, bell peppers, and beef on skewers; alternatively, sprinkle with Black Pepper
- Let it cook for 10 minutes, in a preheated air fryer at 400F, flip halfway through.
- Serve with yogurt dipping sauce.

Nutritional Value: per serving: Calories 268 |Proteins 20g |Carbs 15g|Fat 10g |

1.32 Air Fryer Rotisserie Chicken

(Prep Time: 5 mints| Cook Time: 60 mints| Servings: 6)

Ingredients

- **Paprika:** 1 tsp.
- One chicken
- Dried basil: 1 tsp.
- Onion powder: 1/2 tsp.
- Dried oregano: 1 tsp.
- Pepper: half tsp.
- **Salt:** 1 and 1/2 tsp.
- Chopped cilantro and scallions

Instructions

- Let the air fryer preheat to 360F.
- In a bowl, add all the spices and rub it all over the chicken.
- Put the chicken in the air fryer and let it cook at 360F for half an hour or more, if required.
- Serve with salad greens and top with scallions and cilantro.

Nutritional value: per serving: Calories: 391kcal | Carbohydrates: 1g | Protein: 34g | Fat: 27g

1.33 Air Fryer Hamburger

(Prep Time: 5 mints| Cook Time:13 mints| Servings: 4)

Ingredients

- Buns:4
- Lean ground beef chuck: 4 cups
- **Salt,** to taste
- Slices of any cheese: 4 slices
- Black Pepper, to taste

Instructions

- Let the air fryer preheat to 350 F.
- In a bowl, add lean ground beef, pepper, and salt. Mix well and form patties.
- Put them in the air fryer in one layer only, cook for 6 minutes, flip them halfway through. One minute before you take out the patties add cheese on top.
- When cheese is melted, take out from the air fryer.
- Add ketchup, any dressing to your buns, add tomatoes and lettuce and patties.
- Serve hot.

Nutritional value: per serving: Calories: 520kcal | Carbohydrates: 22g | Protein: 31g | Fat: 34g |

1.34 Lemon-Garlic Chicken Thighs

(Prep Time: 2 hours' mints| Cook Time: 35 mints| Servings: 4)

Ingredients

- Lemon juice ¼ cup

- 1 Tbsp. olive oil
- 1 tsp mustard
- Cloves of garlic
- ¼ tsp salt
- ⅛ tsp black pepper
- Chicken thighs
- Lemon wedges

Instructions

- In a bowl, whisk together the olive oil, lemon juice, mustard Dijon, garlic, salt, and pepper.
- Place the chicken thighs in a large plastic resalable bag. Spill marinade over chicken & seal bag, ensuring all chicken parts are covered. Cool for at least 2 hours.
- Preheat a frying pan to 360 F (175 C).
- Remove the chicken with towels from the marinade, & pat dry.
- Place pieces of chicken in the air fryer basket, if necessary, cook them in batches.
- Fry till chicken is no longer pink on the bone & the juices run smoothly, 22 to 24 min. Upon serving, press a lemon slice across each piece.

Nutritional value: per serving: Cal 258|Fat: 18.6g| Carbs: 3.6g| Protein: 19.4g

1.35 Smothered Chicken Thighs

(Prep Time: 30 mints| Cook Time:30 mints| Servings: 4)

Ingredients

- 8-ounce of chicken thighs
- 1 tsp paprika
- One pinch salt
- Mushrooms: half cup
- Onions, roughly sliced

Instructions

- Let the air fryer preheat to 400F
- Chicken thighs season with paprika, salt, and pepper on both sides.
- Place the thighs in the air fryer and cook for 20 minutes.
- Meanwhile, sauté the mushroom and onion.
- Take out the thighs from the air fryer serve with sautéed mushrooms and onions.
- And serve with chopped scallions and on the side of salad greens

Nutritional value: per serving: Kcal 466.3| Fat: 32g| Net Carbs: 2.4g|Protein: 40.5g

1.36 Garlic Parmesan Chicken Tenders

(Prep Time: 5 mints| Cook Time:12 mints| Servings: 4)

Ingredients

- One egg
- Eight raw chicken tenders
- Water: 2 tablespoons
- Olive oil

To coat

- Panko breadcrumbs: 1 cup
- Half tsp of salt
- Black Pepper: 1/4 teaspoon

- Garlic powder: 1 teaspoon
- Onion powder: 1/2 teaspoon
- Parmesan cheese: 1/4 cup
- any dipping Sauce

Instructions

- Add all the coating ingredients in a big bowl
- In another bowl, mix water and egg.
- Dip the chicken in the egg mix then in the coating mix.
- Put the tenders in the air fry basket in a single layer.
- Spray with the olive oil light
- Cook at 400 degrees for 12 minutes. Flip the chicken halfway through.
- Serve with salad greens and enjoy.

Nutritional value: per serving: Calories: 220kcal | Carbohydrates: 13g | Protein: 27g | Fat: 6g |

1.37 Mixed Vegetables with Chicken

(Prep Time: 20 mints| Cook Time:20 mints| Servings: 2)

Ingredients

- 1/2 onion diced
- Chicken breast: 4 cups, cubed pieces
- Half zucchini chopped
- Italian seasoning: 1 tablespoon
- Bell pepper chopped: 1/2 cup
- Clove of garlic pressed
- Broccoli florets: 1/2 cup
- Olive oil: 2 tablespoons
- Half teaspoon of chili powder, garlic powder, pepper, salt,

Instructions

- Let the air fryer heat to 400 F and dice the vegetables
- In a bowl, add the seasoning, oil and add vegetables, chicken and toss well
- Place chicken and vegetables in the air fryer, and cook for ten minutes, toss half way through, cook in batches.
- Make sure the veggies are charred, and chicken is cooked through.
- Serve hot.

Nutritional value: per serving: :| Calories: 230kcal | Carbohydrates: 8g | Protein: 26g | Fat: 10g |

1.38 Air Fryer Blackened Chicken Breast

(Prep Time: 10 mints| Cook Time:20 mints| Servings: 2)

Ingredients

- Paprika: 2 teaspoons
- Ground thyme: 1 teaspoon
- Cumin: 1 teaspoon
- Cayenne pepper: half tsp.
- Onion powder: half tsp.
- Black Pepper: half tsp.
- Salt: ¼ teaspoon
- Vegetable oil: 2 teaspoons
- Pieces of chicken breast halves (without bones and skin)

Instructions

- In a mixing bowl, add onion powder, salt, cumin, paprika, black pepper, thyme, and cayenne pepper. Mix it well.
- Drizzle oil over chicken and rub. Dip each piece of chicken in blackening spice blend on both sides.
- Let it rest for five minutes while the air fryer is preheating.
- Preheat it for five minutes at 360F.
- Put the chicken in the air fryer and let it cook for ten minutes. Flip and then cook for another ten minutes.
- After, let it sit for five minutes, then slice and serve with the side of green

Nutritional value: per serving: 432.1 calories| protein 79.4g| carbohydrates 3.2g| fat 9.5g

1.39 Mexican-Style Air Fryer Stuffed Chicken Breasts

(Prep Time: 20 mints| Cook Time:10 mints| Servings: 2)

Ingredients

- Olive oil: 2 teaspoons
- One chicken breast (skinless, boneless)
- Chili powder: 4 tsp., divided
- Chipotle flakes: 2 tsp.
- Half bell pepper, sliced
- Mexican oregano: 2 tsp.
- Salt and pepper, to taste
- Ground cumin: 4 tsp., divided
- Half juice of a lime
- Half onion, sliced
- One jalapeno pepper, sliced

Instructions

- In a bowl, add two tsp of cumin and two tsp. of chili powder, mix well
- Let the air fryer Preheat to 400 F
- Pound the chicken breast until 1/4 inch of thickness remains.
- In a bowl, mix remaining chili powder, chipotle flakes, salt, oregano, remaining cumin, and pepper. Rub this spice mix all over the chicken.
- Put half the bell pepper, jalapeno, and onion in the breast half. Roll the chicken around it and secure with large toothpicks.
- Add olive oil on breast rolls and coat in the cumin-chili mixture.
- Add chicken breast to air fryer and cook for six minutes.
- Flip the breast rolls, and cook for five minutes more until the chicken's temperature reaches 165 F.
- Drizzle lime juice on top of breast rolls and serve hot.

Nutritional value: per serving: 185.3 calories| protein 14.8g | carbohydrates 15.2g |fat 8.5g

1.40 Chicken Fajitas

(Prep Time: 10 mints| Cook Time:20 mints| Servings: 6)

Ingredients

- Chicken breasts: 4 cups, cut into thin strips
- Bell peppers, sliced

- Salt: half tsp.
- Cumin: 1 tsp.
- Garlic powder: 1/4 tsp
- Chili powder: half tsp.
- Lime juice: 1 tbsp.

Instructions

- In a bowl, add seasonings, chicken and lime juice, and mix well.
- Then add sliced peppers, and coat well.
- Spray the air fryer with olive oil.
- Put the chicken and peppers in, and cook for 15 minutes at 400 F. flip halfway through.
- Serve with wedges of lemons and enjoy.

Nutritional value: per serving: Calories 140 |Proteins 22g |Carbs 6g|Fat 5g |Fiber 7g

1.41 Air Fryer Sesame Chicken Breast

(Prep Time: 5 mints| Cook Time:30 mints| Servings: 2)

Ingredients

- Sesame oil: 2 Tbsp.
- Chicken breasts: 2 pieces boneless and skin-on
- Black Pepper: 1/2 tsp
- Onions powder: 1 Tbsp.
- Sweet paprika: 1 Tbsp.
- Salt: 1 tsp
- Cayenne pepper: 1/4 tsp
- Granulated garlic: 1 Tbsp.

Instructions

- Pour sesame oil all over chicken and rub, and sprinkle with all spices, pepper, and salt
- Coat the chicken well in spices.
- Put the chicken breasts in the air fryer, skin side up. Make sure to leave space between chicken pieces.
- Cook for 20 minutes, at 380F. After 20 minutes, turn the chicken and cook for ten minutes more.
- Take out from the air fryer and let it rest for five minutes.
- Serve with air-fried vegetables.

Nutritional value: per serving: Calories 240 |Proteins 20g |Carbs 14g |Fat 20g |

1.42 Herb-Marinated Chicken Thighs

(Prep Time: 30 mints| Cook Time:10 mints| Servings: 4)

Ingredients

- Chicken thighs: 8 skin-on, bone-in,
- Lemon juice: 2 Tablespoon
- Onion powder: half teaspoon
- Garlic powder: 2 teaspoon
- Spike Seasoning: 1 teaspoon.
- Olive oil: 1/4 cup
- Dried basil: 1 teaspoon
- Dried oregano: half teaspoon.
- Black Pepper: 1/4 tsp.

Instructions

- In a bowl, add dried oregano, olive oil, lemon juice, dried sage, garlic powder, Spike Seasoning, onion powder, dried basil, black pepper.
- In a zip lock bag, add the spice blend and the chicken and mix well.
- Marinate the chicken in the refrigerator for at least six hours or more.
- Preheat the air fryer to 360F.
- Put the chicken in the air fryer basket, cook for six-eight minutes, flip the chicken, and cook for six minutes more.
- Until the internal chicken temperature reaches 165F.
- Take out from the air fryer and serve with microgreens.

Nutritional value: per serving: Cal 100|Fat: 9g| Carbs 1g|Protein 4g

1.43 Lemon Pepper Chicken

(Prep Time: 3 mints| Cook Time:15 mints| Servings: 2)

Ingredients

- Two Lemons rind, juice, and zest
- One Chicken Breast
- Minced Garlic: 1 Tsp
- Black Peppercorns: 2 tbsp.
- Chicken Seasoning: 1 Tbsp.
- Salt & pepper, to taste

Instructions

- Let the air fryer preheat to 180C.
- In a large aluminum foil, add all the seasonings along with lemon rind.
- Add salt and pepper to chicken and rub the seasonings all over chicken breast.
- Put the chicken in aluminum foil. And fold it tightly.
- Flatten the chicken inside foil with a rolling pin
- Put it in the air fryer and cook at 180 C for 15 minutes.
- Serve hot.

Nutritional value: per serving: Calories: 140 | Carbohydrates: 24g | Protein: 13g | Fat: 2g

1.44 Air Fryer Chicken Parmesan

(Prep Time: 20 mints| Cook Time:30 mints| Servings: 4)

Ingredients

- Whole wheat seasoned breadcrumbs: 6 tbsp.
- Chicken breast: 2 pieces, make four thinner cutlets
- Mozzarella cheese: 6 tbsp. (reduced fat)
- Parmesan cheese: 2 tbsp. (grated)
- Marinara: 1/2 cup
- One tbsp. melted butter
- Olive oil

Instructions

- Let the air fryer preheat to 360 F for three minutes.
- In a bowl, add parmesan cheese and breadcrumbs, mix well.

- Drizzle melted butter on the chicken and coat in the parmesan mixture. Shake excess off.
- Put the chicken in the air fryer and spray with oil.
- Cook for six minutes, flip the chicken over. Add shredded cheese and sauce on top and cook for another three minutes.
- Serve with microgreens.

Nutritional value: per serving: Calories: 251kcal | Carbohydrates: 14g | Protein: 31.5g | Fat: 9.5g

1.45 Air Fryer No Breading Chicken Breast

(Prep Time: 10 mints | Cook Time:20 mints | Servings: 2)

Ingredients

- Olive oil spray
- Chicken breasts: 4 (boneless)
- Onion powder: 3/4 teaspoon
- Salt: ¼ cup
- Smoked paprika: half tsp.
- 1/8 tsp. of cayenne pepper
- Garlic powder: 3/4 teaspoon
- Dried parsley: half tsp.

Instructions

- In a large bowl, add six cups of warm water, add salt (1/4 cup) and mix to dissolve.
- Put chicken breasts to the warm salted water, and let it refrigerate for almost 2 hours.
- Remove from water and pat dry.
- In a bowl, add all the spices with ¾ tsp. of salt. Spray the oil all over the chicken and rub the spice mix all over the chicken.
- Let the air fryer heat at 380F.
- Put the chicken in the air fryer and cook for ten minutes. Flip halfway through and serve with salad green.

Nutritional value: per serving: Calories: 208kcal | Carbohydrates: 1g | Protein: 39g | Fat: 4.5g

1.46 Crispy Parmesan Buttermilk Chicken Tenders

(Prep Time: 10 mints | Cook Time:18 mints | Servings: 4)

Ingredients

- Half cup of all-purpose flour
- Buttermilk: 3/4 cup
- Chicken breasts: 2, boneless, skinless
- Kosher salt: 3/4 teaspoon, divided
- Grated Parmesan cheese: 1/4 cup
- Black Pepper: 3/4 teaspoon, divided
- Worcestershire sauce: 1 and 1/2 teaspoons, divided
- Smoked paprika: half teaspoon, divided
- Oil spray
- Whole wheat breadcrumbs: 1 and 1/2 cups
- One large egg

Instructions

- Cut the chicken into tenders.

- In a bowl, add buttermilk and Worcestershire sauce (half of it), salt, and half
- of paprika and pepper. Add this mix in a zip lock bag with chicken tenders, and let it marinate for six hours or more.
- In a bowl, add melted butter and breadcrumbs, parmesan cheese and combine well
- Whisk the egg with remaining Worcestershire sauce.
- In another bowl, add the smoked paprika, pepper, flour, and salt.
- Coat the tenders in flour mixture, then in egg again, then in breadcrumbs mixture.
- Let the air fryer preheat to 400 F. put the breaded tenders in the air fryer basket in one even layer.
- Cook at 400 F for 13-15 minutes, flip the chicken after half time.
- Serve with sauces and microgreen
- **Nutritional value:** per serving: Calories: 251kcal | Carbohydrates: 14g | Protein: 31.5g | Fat: 9.5g

1.47 Air Fryer Southwest Chicken

(Prep Time: 20 mints | Cook Time:30 mints | Servings: 4)

Ingredients

- Avocado oil: one tbsp.
- Four cups of boneless, skinless, chicken breast
- Chili powder: half tsp.
- Salt, to taste
- Cumin: half tsp.
- Onion powder: 1/4 tsp.
- Lime juice: two tbsp.
- Garlic powder: 1/4 tsp

Instructions

- In a zip lock bag, add chicken, oil, and lime juice.
- Add all spices in a bowl and rub all over the chicken in the zip lock bag.
- Let it marinate in the fridge for ten minutes or more.
- Take chicken out from the zip lock bag and put it in the air fryer.
- Cook for 25 minutes at 400 F, flipping chicken halfway through until internal temperature reaches 165 degrees.

Nutritional value: per serving: Calories: 165kcal | Carbohydrates: 1g | Protein: 24g | Fat: 6g

1.48 Air- Fried Grilled BBQ Chicken

(Prep Time: 10 mints | Cook Time: 12 mints | Servings: 2)

Ingredients

- Chicken Steaks: 2 pieces
- Sea salt: 1 tsp.
- 1 tsp. olive oil
- Freshly ground Black Pepper: 1/2 teaspoon

Blue Cheese &Butter

- Blue Cheese: 1/ 4 cup
- 1/2 cup of butter (at room temperature)

Instructions

- While making steak, the most important thing is to let the meat rest at

  temperature for 30 minutes, for the minimum.
- Start the recipe by letting the air fryer heat. For making any kind of steak, you should always preheat the air fryer. Therefore, the meat would come out well, then turn the air fryer on at 400 F for 5 minutes.
- Rub the steak with butter or herb-infused olive oil and sprinkle with sea salt and black pepper.
- Place the stakes for 6 minutes in the air fryer, then turn over again for almost 6 minutes.
- Yet again, rest the steak for the very least for 5 minutes, and then slice it.
- The steaks will keep on cooking, even after it is done cooking.
- Only combine the butter and the Blue Cheese in a small bowl to mix to make the cheese. You can serve the steak as you like.
- Put the butter in a wrap and rolled it tightly, it would appear like a roll, keep it refrigerated, and cut off a few bits for each portion.

Nutritional value: per serving: Calories 200 | Proteins 20g | Carbs 2g | Fat 5g |

1.49 Bell Peppers Frittata

(Prep time: 10 min | Cooking time: 20 min | Servings: 4)

Ingredients

- 2 Tablespoons olive oil
- 2 cups chicken sausage, casings removed and chopped
- One sweet onion, chopped
- 1 red bell pepper, chopped
- 1 orange bell pepper, chopped
- 1 green bell pepper, chopped
- Salt and black pepper to taste
- 8 eggs, whisked
- ½ cup mozzarella cheese, shredded
- 2 teaspoons oregano, chopped

Instructions

- Add 1 spoonful of oil to the air fryer, add bacon, heat to 320 degrees F, and brown for 1 minute.
- Remove remaining butter, onion, red bell pepper, orange and white, mix and simmer for another 2 minutes.
- Stir and cook for 15 minutes, add oregano, salt, pepper, and eggs.
- Add mozzarella, leave frittata aside for a couple of minutes, divide and serve between plates.
- Enjoy.

Nutritional value: per serving: calories 212, fat 4g, fiber 6g, carbs 8g, protein 12g

1.50. Mushroom Oatmeal

(Prep time: 10 min | Cooking time: 20 min | Servings: 4)

Ingredients

- One small yellow onion, chopped
- 1 cup steel-cut oats

- 1 Garlic cloves, minced
- 2 Tablespoons butter
- ½ cup of water
- One and a half cup of canned chicken stock
- Thyme springs, chopped
- 2 Tablespoons extra virgin olive oil
- ½ cup gouda cheese, grated
- 1 cup mushroom, sliced
- Salt and black pepper to taste

Instructions

- Heat a pan over medium heat, which suits your air fryer with the butter, add

  onions and garlic, stir and cook for 4 minutes.
- Add oats, sugar, salt, pepper, stock, and thyme, stir, place in the air fryer and cook for 16 minutes at 360 degrees F.
- In the meantime, prepare a skillet over medium heat with the olive oil, add mushrooms, cook them for 3 minutes, add oatmeal and cheese, whisk, divide into bowls and serve for breakfast.
- Enjoy.

Nutritional value: per serving: calories 284|fat 8g| fiber 8g|carbs 20g| protein 17g

1.51 Green Bean Casserole

(Prep time: 10 min| Cook Time: 15 min | Serves 4)

Ingredients

- 4 tablespoons unsalted butter
- 1/4 cup diced yellow onion
- 1/2 cup chopped white mushrooms
- 1/2 cup heavy whipping cream
- ¼ cup low-fat cream cheese
- 1/2 cup chicken broth
- 1/4 teaspoon xanthan gum
- 4 cups fresh green beans, edges trimmed
- 1 tbsp. of pork rinds, finely ground

Instructions

- Melt butter in a medium saucepan over low heat. Sauté the onion and mushrooms for around 3–5 minutes, before they become soft and fragrant.
- Apply hard cream whipping, cream cheese, and broth to the saucepan. Whisk easily before. Bring to a boil, then diminish to a simmer. Sprinkle the xanthan gum into the pan and cook up.
- Cut the green beans into 2 "pieces and put them in a 4-cup circular baking dish. Spill the sauce mixture over them and stir until cooked. Cover the bowl with the rinds of the ground pork.
- Set the temperature to 320 ° F and change the timer for 15 minutes.
- Top when fully baked, golden and green beans fork tender. Serve soft.

Nutritional value: per serving: calories: 267|protein: 3.6 g| fiber: 3.2 g| net carbohydrates: 6.5 g| fat: 23.4 g| |

Chapter 2: Optavia Lean & Green Low Budget Recipes

2.1 Air Fryer Sweet & Sour Chicken

(Prep Time: 5 mints | Cook Time: 10 mints | Servings: 2)

Ingredients

Chicken

- 4 cups chicken breasts /thighs: cut into one-inch pieces
- Cornstarch: 2 tablespoons

Sweet & Sour Sauce

- Cornstarch: 2 tablespoons
- Pineapple juice: 1 cup
- Water: 2 tablespoons
- Honey: half cup
- Soy sauce: 1 tablespoon
- Rice wine vinegar: 3 tablespoons
- Ground ginger: 1/4 teaspoon

Optional

- 1/4 cup pineapple chunks
- 3-4 drops of red food coloring (for traditional orange look)

Instructions

- Let the air fryer preheat to 400 degrees.
- Coat the chicken in cornstarch, until the chicken is coated completely.
- Put the chicken in the air fryer and let it cook for 7,9 minutes. Take out from air fryer
- In the meantime, in a saucepan, add pineapple juice, ginger, brown sugar, soy sauce, and rice wine vinegar and cook. Let it simmer for five minutes.
- Make cornstarch slurry and add in the sauce. Let it simmer for one minute.
- Coat cooked chicken pieces and serve with steamed vegetables

Nutritional value: per serving: Cal 302|Fat: 8g| Carbs 18g|Protein 22g

2.2 Air Fryer Buffalo Cauliflower

(Prep Time: 5 mints | Cook Time:15 mints | Servings: 4)

Ingredients

- Homemade buffalo sauce: 1/2 cup
- One head of cauliflower, cut bite-size pieces
- Butter melted: 1 tablespoon
- Olive oil
- Kosher salt & pepper, to taste

Instructions

- Spray cooking oil on the air fryer basket.
- In a bowl, add buffalo sauce, melted butter, pepper, and salt. Mix well.
- Put the cauliflower bits in the air fryer and spray the olive oil over it. Let it cook at 400 F for 7 minutes.
- Remove the cauliflower from the air fryer and add it to the sauce. Coat the cauliflower well.
- Put the sauce coated cauliflower back into the air fryer.

- Cook at 400 F, for 7-8 minutes or until crispy.
- Take out from the air fryer and serve with leaner protein.

Nutritional value: per serving: Calories 101kcal | Carbohydrates 4g | Protein 3g | Fat: 7g

2.3 Low Carb Air-Fried Calzones

(Prep Time: 15 mints| Cook Time:27 mints| Servings: 2)

Ingredients

- Cooked chicken breast: 1/3 cup(shredded)
- One teaspoon olive oil
- Spinach leaves(baby): 3 cups
- Whole-wheat pizza dough, freshly prepared
- Marinara sauce: 1/3 cup(lower-sodium)
- Diced red onion:1/4 cup
- Skim mozzarella cheese: 6 Tbsp.
- Cooking spray

Instructions

- In a medium skillet, over a medium flame, add oil, onions. Sauté until soft. Then add spinach leaves, cook until wilted. Turn off the heat and add chicken and marinara sauce.
- Cut the dough into two pieces.
- Add 1/4 of the spinach mix on each circle dough piece.
- Add skim shredded cheese on top. Fold the dough over and crimp the edges.
- Spray the calzones with cooking spray.
- Put calzones in the air fryer. Cook for 12 minutes, at 325°F until dough is light brown. Turn the calzone over and cook for eight more minutes.

Nutritional value: per serving: Calories 348|Fat 12g | Protein 21g |Carbohydrate 18g

2.4 Air Fryer Low Carb Chicken Bites

(Prep Time: 10 mints| Cook Time:10 mints| Servings: 3)

Ingredients

- Chicken breast: 2 cups
- Kosher salt& pepper to taste
- Smashed potatoes: one cup
- Scallions: ¼ cup
- One Egg beat
- Whole wheat breadcrumbs: 1 cup

Instructions

- Boil the chicken until soft.
- Shred the chicken with the help of a fork.
- Add the smashed potatoes, scallions to the shredded chicken. Season with kosher salt and pepper.
- Coat with egg and then in bread crumbs.
- Put in the air fryer, and cook for 8 minutes at 380F. Or until golden brown.
- Serve warm.

Nutritional value: per serving: Calories: 234 | protein 25g | carbs 15g | fat 9 g

2.5 Air Fryer Popcorn Chicken

(Prep Time: 10 mints | Cook Time:20 mints | Servings: 2)

Ingredients

For Marinade

- 8 cups, chicken tenders, cut into bite-size pieces
- Freshly ground black pepper: 1/2 tsp
- **Almond milk:** 2 cups
- Salt: 1 tsp
- paprika: 1/2 tsp

Dry Mix

- Salt: 3 tsp
- Flour: 3 cups
- Paprika: 2 tsp
- Oil spray
- Freshly ground black pepper: 2 tsp

Instructions

- In a bowl, add all marinade ingredients and chicken. Mix well, and put it in a Zip lock bag and refrigerator for two hours for the minimum, or six hours.
- In a large bowl, add all the dry ingredients.
- Coat the marinated chicken to the dry mix. Into the marinade again then for the second time in the dry mixture.
- Spray the air fryer basket with olive oil and place the breaded chicken pieces in one single layer. Spray oil over the chicken pieces too.
- Cook at 370 degrees for 10 minutes, tossing halfway through.
- Serve immediately with salad greens or dipping sauce.

Nutritional value: per serving: Calories 340 | Proteins 20g | Carbs 14g | Fat 10g |

2.6 Air Fried Cheesy Chicken Omelet

(Prep Time: 5 mints | Cook Time: 18 mints | Servings: 2)

Ingredients

- Cooked Chicken Breast: half cup(diced)divided
- Four eggs
- Onion powder: 1/4 tsp, divided
- Salt: 1/2 tsp., divided
- Pepper: 1/4 tsp., divided
- Shredded cheese: 2 tbsp. divided
- Granulated garlic: 1/4 tsp, divided

Instructions

- Take two ramekins, grease with olive oil.
- Add two eggs in each ramekin. Add cheese with seasoning.
- Blend to combine. Add 1/4 cup of cooked chicken on top.
- Cook for 14-18 minutes, in the air fryer at 330 F, or until fully cooked.

Nutritional value: per serving: Calories 185 | Proteins 20g | Carbs 10g | Fat 5g |

2.7 Air-Fried Tortilla Hawaiian Pizza

(Prep Time: 10 mints| Cook Time:20 mints| Servings: 1)

Ingredients

- Mozzarella Cheese
- Tortilla wrap
- Tomato sauce: 1 tbsp.
- Toppings
- Cooked chicken shredded or hotdog: 2 tbsp.
- Pineapple pieces: 3 tbsp.
- Ham: half slice, cut into pieces
- Cheese slice cut into pieces

Instructions

- Lay tortilla flat on a plate, add tomato sauce and spread it.
- Add some shredded mozzarella, add toppings. Top with cheese slices
- Put in the air fryer and cook for five or ten minutes at 160 C.
- Take out from the air fryer and slice it. Serve hot with baby spinach.

Nutritional value: per serving: Calories 178 |Proteins 21g |Carbs 15g |Fat 15g |

2.8 Air Fryer Personal Mini Pizza

(Prep Time: 2 mints| Cook Time:5 mints| Servings: 1)

Ingredients

- Sliced olives: 1/4 cup
- One pita bread
- One tomato
- Shredded cheese: 1/2 cup

Instructions

- Let the air fryer preheat to 350 F
- Lay pita flat on a plate. Add cheese, slices of tomatoes, and olives.
- Cook for five minutes at 350 F
- Take the pizza out of the air fryer.
- Slice it and enjoy

Nutritional value: per serving: Calories: 344kcal | Carbohydrates: 37g | Protein: 18g | Fat: 13g |

2.9 Air Fryer Party Meatballs

(Prep Time: 5 mints| Cook Time:15 mints| Servings: 4)

Ingredients

- Worcester Sauce: 21/2 Tbsp.
- Lean Mince Beef: 4 cups
- Dry Mustard: half tsp.
- Tabasco: 1 Tbsp.
- Brown Sugar; half cup
- Vinegar: ¼ Cup
- Tomato Ketchup: ¾ Cup
- Lemon Juice: 1 Tbsp.
- Three crushed Gingersnaps

Instructions

- Add all seasoning ingredients in a large bowl and mix well.
- Then add minced beef and mix well.
- With your hands, make them into medium sized balls.

- Put them into the air fryer and cook at 375F for 15 minutes, until cooked through completely.
- Take them out, and add sticks to them before serving.

Nutritional value: per serving: Calories: 383kcal | Carbohydrates: 25g | Protein: 22g | Fat: 13g

2.10 Air Fryer Chicken Nuggets

(Prep Time: 15 mints| Cook Time:15 mints| Servings: 4)

Ingredients

- Olive oil spray
- Skinless boneless: 2 chicken breasts, cut into bite pieces
- Half tsp. of kosher salt& freshly ground black pepper, to taste
- Grated parmesan cheese: 2 tablespoons
- Italian seasoned breadcrumbs: 6 tablespoons (whole wheat)
- Whole wheat breadcrumbs: 2 tablespoons
- olive oil: 2 teaspoons

Instructions

- Let the air fryer preheat for 8 minutes, to 400 F
- In a big mixing bowl, add panko, parmesan cheese, and breadcrumbs and mix well.
- Sprinkle kosher salt and pepper on chicken and olive oil, mix well.
- Take a few pieces of chicken, dunk them to breadcrumbs mixture.
- Put these pieces in an air fryer and spray with olive oil.
- Cook for 8 minutes, turning halfway through
- Enjoy with kale chips.

Nutritional value: per serving: Calories: 188kcal, Carbohydrates: 8g, Protein: 25g, Fat: 4.5g

2.11 5-Ingredient Air Fryer Lemon Chicken

(Prep Time: 5 mints| Cook Time:15 mints| Servings: 4)

Ingredients

- Whole-wheat crumbs: 1 and 1/2 cups
- Six pieces of chicken tenderloins
- Two eggs
- Two half lemons and lemon slices
- Kosher salt to taste

Instructions

- In a dish, whisk the eggs.
- In a separate dish, add the breadcrumbs
- With egg, coat the chicken and roll in breadcrumbs.
- Add the breaded chicken in the air fryer
- Cook for 14 minutes at 400 F, flip the chicken halfway through.
- Take out from air fryer and squeeze lemon juice and sprinkle with kosher salt and serve with lemon slices.

Nutritional value: per serving: Cal 240| Fat: 12g| Net Carbs: 13g|Protein: 27g

2.12 Low Carb Chicken Tenders

(Prep Time: 10 mints| Cook Time:20 mints| Servings: 3)

Ingredients

- Chicken tenderloins: 4 cups
- Eggs: one
- Superfine Almond Flour: ½ cup
- Powdered Parmesan cheese: ½ cup
- Kosher Sea salt: ½ teaspoon
- (1-teaspoon) freshly ground black pepper
- (1/2 teaspoon) Cajun seasoning,

Instructions

- On a small plate, pour the beaten egg.
- Mix all ingredients in a zip lock bag the cheese. Almond flour freshly ground black pepper & kosher salt and other seasonings.
- Spray the air fryer with oil spray.
- To avoid clumpy fingers with breading and egg. Use different hands for egg and breading. Dip each tender in egg and then in bread until they are all breaded.
- Using a fork to place one tender at a time. Bring it in the zip lock bag and shake the bag forcefully. make sure all the tenders are covered in almond mixture
- Using the fork to take out the tender and place it in your air fryer basket.
- Spray oil on the tenders.
- Cook for 12 minutes at 350F, or before 160F registers within. Raise temperature to 400F to shade the surface for 3 minutes.
- Serve with sauce.

Nutritional value: per serving: Calories 280 |Proteins 20g |Carbs 6g|Fat 10g |Fiber 5g

2.13 Cheesy Cauliflower Tots

(Prep Time: 15 mints| Cook Time:12 mints| Servings: 4)

Ingredients

- 1 large head cauliflower
- 1 cup shredded mozzarella cheese
- 1/2 cup grated Parmesan cheese
- 1 large egg
- 1/4 teaspoon garlic powder
- 1/4 teaspoon dried parsley
- 1/8 teaspoon onion powder

Instructions

- Fill a big pot with 2 cups of water on the stovetop, and insert a steamer in the oven. Put to boil bath.
- Break the cauliflower into flower and placed on a steamer box—cover pot and lid.
- Let steam the cauliflower for 7 minutes until the fork-tender. Put in the cheesecloth or clean kitchen towel from the steamer basket and let it cool.
- Push on the sink to eliminate as much extra humidity as possible. If not all of the moisture is removed, the mixture will be too soft to form into tots.

- Mash down to a smooth consistency with a blade.
- In a large mixing bowl, put the cauliflower and add the mozzarella, parmesan, egg, garlic powder, parsley, and onion powder. Remove until well combined. The blend should be smooth but easy to mold.
- Take 2 tablespoons of the mixture and roll the mixture into a tot form. Repeat with mixture leftover. Put the basket into the air fryer.
- Set the temperature to 320 ° F and adjust the timer for 12 minutes.
- Turn the tots halfway through the period of cooking.
- Cauliflower tots should be golden when fully cooked. Serve warm.

Nutritional Value: per serving: calories: 181 | protein 13.5g | fiber 3.0g | carbohydrates: 6.6 g | fat: 9.5 g |

2.14 Tasty Kale & Celery Crackers

(Prep time: 10 min | Cooking time: 20 min | Servings: 6)

Ingredients

- **One** cups flax seed, ground
- 1 cups flax seed, soaked overnight and drained
- 2 bunches kale, chopped
- 1 bunch basil, chopped
- ½ bunch celery, chopped
- 2 garlic cloves, minced
- 1/3 cup olive oil

Instructions

- Mix the ground flaxseed with the celery, kale, basil, and garlic in your food

  processor and mix well.
- Add the oil and soaked flaxseed, then mix again, scatter in the pan of your air fryer, break into medium crackers and cook for 20 minutes at 380 degrees F.
- Serve as an appetizer and break into cups.
- Enjoy

Nutritional Value: per serving: calories 143 | fat 1g | fiber 2g | carbs 8g | Protein 4g

Chapter 3: Optavia Lean & Green Pork Air-fry Recipes

3.1 Low Carb Pork Dumplings with Dipping Sauce

(Prep Time: 30 mints| Cook Time:20 mints| Servings: 6)

Ingredients

- 18 dumpling wrappers
- One teaspoon olive oil
- Bok choy: 4 cups(chopped)
- Rice vinegar: 2 tablespoons
- Diced ginger: 1 tablespoon
- Crushed red pepper: 1/4 teaspoon
- Diced garlic: 1 tablespoon
- Lean ground pork: half cup
- Cooking spray
- Lite soy sauce: 2 teaspoons
- Honey: half tsp.
- Toasted sesame oil: 1 teaspoon
- Finely chopped scallions

Instructions

- In a large skillet, heat olive oil, add bok choy, cook for 6 minutes, and add garlic, ginger, and cook for one minute. Move this mixture on a paper towel and pat dry, excess oil
- In a bowl, add bok choy mixture, crushed red pepper, and lean ground pork and mix well.
- Lay a dumpling wrapper on a plate and add one tbsp. of filling in the wrapper's middle. With water, seal the edges and crimp it.
- Air spray the air fryer basket, add dumplings in the air fryer basket, and cook at 375 F for 12 minutes or until browned.
- In the meantime, to make the sauce, add sesame oil, rice vinegar, scallions, soy sauce, and honey in a bowl mix together.
- Serve the dumplings with sauce.

Nutritional value: per serving: Calories 140| Fat 5g |Protein 12g |Carbohydrate 9g|

3.2 Air Fryer Pork Taquitos

(Prep Time: 10 mints| Cook Time:20 mints| Servings: 10)

Ingredients

- Pork tenderloin: 3 cups, cooked & shredded
- Cooking spray
- Shredded mozzarella: 2 and 1/2 cups, fat-free
- 10 small tortillas
- Salsa for dipping
- One juice of a lime

Instructions

- Let the air fryer preheat to 380 F
- Add lime juice to pork and mix well
- With a damp towel over the tortilla, microwave for ten seconds to soften

- Add pork filling and cheese on top, in a tortilla, roll up the tortilla tightly.
- Place tortillas on a greased foil pan
- Spray oil over tortillas. Cook for 7-10 minutes or until tortillas is golden brown, flip halfway through.
- Serve with salad greens.

Nutritional value: per serving: Cal 253 |Fat: 18g| Carbs: 10g| Protein: 20g|

3.3 Gluten-Free Air Fryer Chicken Fried Brown Rice

(Prep Time: 10 mints| Cook Time:20 mints| Servings: 2)

Ingredients

- Olive Oil Cooking Spray
- Chicken Breast: 1 Cup, Diced & Cooked &
- White Onion: 1/4 cup chopped
- Celery: 1/4 Cup chopped
- Cooked brown rice: 4 Cups
- Carrots: 1/4 cup chopped

Instructions

- Place foil on the air fryer basket, make sure to leave room for air to flow, roll up on the sides
- Spray with olive oil, the foil. Mix all ingredients.
- On top of the foil, add all ingredients in the air fryer basket.
- Give an olive oil spray on the mixture.
- Cook for five minutes at 390F.
- Open the air fryer and give a toss to the mixture
- cook for five more minutes at 390F.
- Take out from air fryer and serve hot.

Nutritional value: per serving: Cal 350|Fat: 6g|Carbs 20g|Protein 22g

3.4 Air Fryer Whole Wheat Crusted Pork Chops

(Prep Time: 10 mints| Cook Time:12 mints| Servings: 4)

Ingredients

- Whole-wheat breadcrumbs: 1 cup
- Salt: ¼ teaspoon
- Pork chops: 2-4 pieces (center cut and boneless)
- Chili powder: half teaspoon
- Parmesan cheese: 1 tablespoon
- Paprika: 1½ teaspoons
- One egg beaten
- Onion powder: half teaspoon
- Granulated garlic: half teaspoon
- Pepper, to taste

Instructions

- Let the air fryer preheat to 400 F
- rub kosher salt on each side of pork chops, let it rest
- Add beaten egg in a big bowl
- Add Parmesan cheese, breadcrumbs, garlic, pepper, paprika, chili powder, and onion powder in a bowl and mix well
- Dip pork chop in egg then in breadcrumb mixture
- Put it in the air fryer and spray with oil.

- Let it cook for 12 minutes at 400 F. flip it over, halfway through. Cook for another six minutes.
- Serve with salad greens.

Nutritional value: per serving: 425 calories | 20 g fat | 5 g fiber | 31 g protein | Carbs

19 g

3.5 Air Fryer Pork Chop & Broccoli

(Prep Time: 20 mints | Cook Time:20 mints | Servings: 2)

Ingredients

- Broccoli florets: 2 cups
- Bone-in pork chop: 2 pieces
- Paprika: half tsp.
- Avocado oil: 2 tbsp.
- Garlic powder: half tsp.
- Onion powder: half tsp.
- Two cloves of crushed garlic
- Salt: 1 teaspoon divided

Instructions

- Let the air fryer preheat to 350 degrees. Spray the basket with cooking oil
- Add one tbsp. Oil, onion powder, half tsp. of salt, garlic powder, and paprika in a bowl mix well, rub this spice mix to the pork chop's sides
- Add pork chops in air fryer basket and let it cook for five minutes
- In the meantime, add one tsp. oil, garlic, half tsp of salt, and broccoli to a bowl and coat well
- Flip the pork chop and add the broccoli, let it cook for five more minutes.
- Take out from the air fryer and serve.

Nutritional value: per serving: Calories 483 | Total Fat 20g | Carbohydrates 12g | protein 23 g

3.6 Air Fryer Cheesy Pork Chops

(Prep Time: 5mints | Cook Time:8 mints | Servings: 2)

Ingredients

- 4 lean pork chops
- Salt: half tsp.
- Garlic powder: half tsp.
- Shredded cheese: 4 tbsp.
- Chopped cilantro

Instructions

- Let the air fryer preheat to 350 degrees.
- With garlic, cilantro, and salt, rub the pork chops. Put in the air fryer. Let it cook for four minutes. Flip them and cook for two minutes more.
- Add cheese on top of them and cook for another two minutes or until the cheese is melted.
- Serve with salad greens.

Nutritional value: per serving: Calories: 467kcal | Protein: 61g | Fat: 22g | Saturated Fat: 8g |

3.7 Mustard Glazed Air Fryer Pork Tenderloin

(Prep Time: 10 mints| Cook Time:18 mints| Servings: 4)

Ingredients

- Yellow mustard: ¼ cup
- One pork tenderloin
- Salt: ¼ tsp
- Honey: 3 Tbsp.
- Freshly ground black pepper: ⅛ tsp
- Minced garlic: 1 Tbsp.
- Dried rosemary: 1 tsp
- Italian seasoning: 1 tsp

Instructions

- With a knife, cut the top of pork tenderloin. Add garlic(minced)in the cuts. Then sprinkle with kosher salt and pepper.
- In a bowl, add honey, mustard, rosemary, and Italian seasoning mix until combined. Rub this mustard mix all over pork.
- Let it marinate in the refrigerator for at least two hours.
- Put pork tenderloin in the air fryer basket. Cook for 18-20 minutes at 400 F. with an instant-read thermometer internal temperature of pork should be 145 F
- Take out from the air fryer and serve with a side of salad greens.

Nutritional value: per serving: Calories: 390 | Carbohydrates: 11g | Protein: 59g | Fat: 11g |

3.8 Air Fried Jamaican Jerk Pork Recipe

(Prep Time: 10 mints| Cook Time:20 mints| Servings: 4)

Ingredients

- Pork, cut into three-inch pieces
- **Jerk paste:** ¼ cup

Instructions

- Rub jerk paste all over the pork pieces.
- Let it marinate for four hours, at least, in the refrigerator. Or for more time.
- Let the air fryer preheat to 390 F. spray with olive oil
- Before putting in the air fryer, let the meat sit for 20 minutes at room temperature.
- Cook for 20 minutes at 390 F in the air fryer, flip halfway through.
- Take out from the air fryer let it rest for ten minutes before slicing.
- Serve with microgreens.

Nutritional value: per serving: Calories: 234kcal | Protein: 31g | Fat: 9g |carbs 12 g

3.9 Pork Rind Nachos

(Prep time: 5 min| Cooking Time: 5 min| Serves 2)

Ingredients

- 2 tbsp. of pork rinds
- 1/4 cup shredded cooked chicken
- 1/2 cup shredded Monterey jack cheese
- 1/4 cup sliced pickled jalapeños

- 1/4 cup guacamole
- 1/4 cup full-fat sour cream

Instructions

- Put pork rinds in a 6 "round baking pan. Fill with grilled chicken and Monterey cheese jack. Place the pan in the basket with the air fryer.
- Set the temperature to 370 ° F and set the timer for 5 minutes or until the cheese has been melted.
- Eat right away with jalapeños, guacamole, and sour cream.

Nutritional value: per serving: calories 295 |protein: 30.1 g| fiber: 1.2 g| net carbohydrates: 1.8 g |fat: 27.5 g| carbohydrates: 3.0 g |

Chapter 4: Optavia Lean & Green Turkey Air-fry recipes

4.1 Air Fryer Turkey Fajitas Platter

(Prep Time: 5 mints | Cook Time:20 mints | Servings: 2)

Ingredients

- Cooked Turkey Breast: 1/4 cup
- Six Tortilla Wraps
- One Avocado
- One Yellow Pepper
- One Red Pepper
- Half Red Onion
- Soft Cheese: 5 Tbsp.
- Mexican Seasoning: 2 Tbsp.
- Cumin: 1 Tsp
- Kosher salt& Pepper
- Cajun Spice: 3 Tbsp.
- Fresh Coriander

Instructions

- Chop up the avocado, and slice the vegetables.
- Dice up turkey breast into small bite-size pieces.
- In a bowl, add onions, turkey, soft cheese, and peppers along with seasonings. Mix it well.
- Place it in foil and the air fryer.
- Cook for 20 minutes at 200C.
- Serve hot.

Nutritional value: per serving: Calories: 379kcal | Carbohydrates: 84g | Protein: 30g | Fat: 39g |

4.2 Air Fryer Turkey Breast Tenderloin

(Prep Time: 5 mints | Cook Time:25 mints | Servings: 3)

Ingredients

- Turkey breast tenderloin: one-piece
- Thyme: half tsp.
- Sage: half tsp.
- Paprika: half tsp.
- Pink salt: half tsp.
- Freshly ground black pepper: half tsp.
- **Instructions**
- Let the air fryer preheat to 350 F
- In a bowl, mix all the spices and herbs, rub it all over the turkey.
- Spray oil on the air fryer basket. Put the turkey in the air fryer and let it cook at 350 F for 25 minutes, flip halfway through.
- Serve with micro green salad.

Nutritional value: per serving: Calories: 162kcal | Carbohydrates: 1g | Protein: 13g | Fat: 1g |

4.3 Air-Fried Turkey Breast with Maple Mustard Glaze

(Prep Time: 10 mints | Cook Time:55 mints | Servings: 6)

Ingredients

- Whole turkey breast: 5 pounds

- Olive oil: 2 tsp.
- Maple syrup: 1/4 cup
- Dried sage: half tsp.
- Smoked paprika: half tsp.
- Dried thyme: one tsp.
- Salt: one tsp.
- Freshly ground black pepper: half tsp.
- Dijon mustard: 2 tbsp.

Instructions

- Let the air fryer preheat to 350 F
- Rub the olive oil all over the turkey breast
- In a bowl, mix salt, sage, pepper, thyme, and paprika. Mix well and coat turkey in this spice rub.
- Place the turkey in an air fryer, cook for 25 minutes at 350°F. Flip the turkey over and cook for another 12 minutes. Flip again and cook for another ten minutes. With an instant-read thermometer, the internal temperature should reach 165°F.
- In the meantime, in a saucepan, mix mustard, maple syrup, and with one tsp. of butter.
- Brush this glaze all over the turkey when cooked.
- Cook again for five minutes. Slice and Serve with salad green.

Nutritional value: per serving: Cal 379 | Fat: 23 g| Carbs: 21g | Protein: 52g

4.4 Juicy Turkey Burgers with Zucchini

(Prep Time: 10 mints| Cook Time:10 mints| Servings: 5)

Ingredients

- Gluten-free breadcrumbs: 1/4 cup(seasoned)
- Grated zucchini: 1 cup
- Red onion: 1 tbsp. (grated)
- Lean ground turkey: 4 cups
- One clove of minced garlic
- 1 tsp of kosher salt and fresh pepper

Instructions

- In a bowl, add zucchini (moisture removed with a paper towel), ground turkey, garlic, salt, onion, pepper, breadcrumbs. Mix well
- With your hands makes five patties. But not too thick.
- Let the air fryer preheat to 375 F
- Put in an air fryer in a single layer and cook for 7 minutes or more. Until cooked through and browned.
- Place in buns with ketchup and lettuce and enjoy.

Nutritional value: per serving: Calories: 161kcal|Carbohydrates: 4.5g| Protein: 18g|Fat: 7g|

4.5 Air Fryer Turkey Breast

(Prep Time: 5 mints| Cook Time:55 mints| Servings: 10)

Ingredients

- Turkey breast: 4 pounds, ribs removed, bone with skin

- Olive oil: 1 tablespoon
- Salt: 2 teaspoons
- Dry turkey seasoning (without salt): half tsp.

Instructions

- Rub half tbsp. Of olive oil over turkey breast. Sprinkle salt, turkey seasoning on both sides of turkey breast with half tbsp. Of olive oil.
- Let the air fryer preheat at 350 F. put turkey skin side down in air fryer and cook for 20 minutes, until the turkey's temperature reaches 160 F for half an hour to 40 minutes.
- Let it sit for ten minutes before slicing.
- Serve with salad green.

Nutritional value: per serving: Calories: 226kcal| Protein: 32.5g|Fat: 10g|carbs 22 g

Chapter 5: Optavia Lean & Green Seafood Air-fry Recipes

5.1 Shrimp Spring Rolls

(Prep Time: 10 mints| Cook Time:25 mints| Servings: 4)

Ingredients

- Deveined raw shrimp: half cup chopped(peeled)
- Olive oil: 2 and 1/2 tbsp.
- Matchstick carrots: 1 cup
- Slices of red bell pepper: 1 cup
- Red pepper: 1/4 teaspoon(crushed)
- Slices of snow peas: 3/4 cup
- Shredded cabbage: 2 cups
- Lime juice: 1 tablespoon
- Sweet chili sauce: half cup
- Fish sauce: 2 teaspoons
- Eight spring roll(wrappers)

Instructions

- In a skillet, add one and a half tbsp. of olive, until smoking lightly. Stir in bell pepper, cabbage, carrots, and cook for two minutes. Turn off the heat, take out in a dish and cool for five minutes.
- In a bowl, add shrimp, lime juice, cabbage mixture, crushed red pepper, fish sauce, and snow peas. Mix well
- Lay spring roll wrappers on a plate. Add 1/4 cup of filling in the middle of each wrapper. Fold tightly with water. Brush the olive oil over folded rolls.
- Put spring rolls in the air fryer basket and cook for 6 to 7 minutes at 390°F until light brown and crispy.
- You may serve with sweet chili sauce.

Nutritional value: per serving: Calories 180 |Fat 9g| Protein 17g |Carbohydrate 9g

5.2 Air Fryer Scallops with Tomato Cream Sauce

(Prep Time: 5 mints| Cook Time:10 mints| Servings: 2)

Ingredients

- Sea scallops eight jumbo
- Tomato Paste: 1 tbsp.
- Chopped fresh basil one tablespoon
- 3/4 cup of low-fat Whipping Cream
- Kosher salt half teaspoon
- Ground Freshly black pepper half teaspoon
- Minced garlic 1 teaspoon
- Frozen Spinach, thawed half cup
- Oil Spray

Instructions

- Take a seven-inch pan(heatproof) and add spinach in a single layer at the bottom
- Rub olive oil on both sides of scallops, season with kosher salt and pepper.
- on top of the spinach, place the seasoned scallops
- Put the pan in the air fryer and cook for ten minutes at 350F, until scallops are cooked completely, and internal temperature reaches 135F.

- Serve immediately.

Nutritional value: per serving: Calories: 259kcal | Carbohydrates: 6g | Protein: 19g | Fat: 13g |

5.3 Sriracha & Honey Tossed Calamari

(Prep Time: 10 mints| Cook Time:20 mints| Servings: 2)

Ingredients

- Club soda: 1 cup
- Sriracha: 1-2 Tbsp.
- Calamari tubes: 2 cups
- Flour: 1 cup
- Pinches of salt, freshly ground black pepper, red pepper flakes, and red pepper
- Honey: 1/2 cup

Instructions

- Cut the calamari tubes into rings. Submerge them with club soda. Let it rest for ten minutes.
- In the meantime, in a bowl, add freshly ground black pepper, flour, red pepper, and kosher salt and mix well.
- Drain the calamari and pat dry with a paper towel. Coat well the calamari in the
- flour mix and set aside.
- Spray oil in the air fryer basket and put calamari in one single layer.
- Cook at 375 for 11 minutes. Toss the rings twice while cooking. Meanwhile, to make sauce honey, red pepper flakes, and sriracha in a bowl, well.
- Take calamari out from the basket, mix with sauce cook for another two minutes more. Serve with salad green.

Nutritional value: per serving: Cal 252 | Fat: 38g| Carbs: 3.1g|Protein: 41g

5.4 Air Fryer Southern Style Catfish with Green Beans

(Prep Time: 10 mints| Cook Time:20 mints| Servings: 2)

Ingredients

- Catfish fillets: 2 pieces
- Green beans: half cup, trimmed
- Honey: 2 teaspoon
- Freshly ground black pepper and salt, to taste divided
- Crushed red pepper: half tsp.
- Flour: 1/4 cup
- One egg, lightly beaten
- Dill pickle relish: 3/4 teaspoon
- Apple cider vinegar: half tsp
- 1/3 cup whole-wheat breadcrumbs
- Mayonnaise: 2 tablespoons
- Dill
- Lemon wedges

Instructions

- In a bowl, add green beans, spray them cooking oil. Coat with crushed red pepper, 1/8 teaspoon of kosher salt, and half tsp. Of honey and cook in the air fryer at 400 F until soft and browned, for 12 minutes. Take out from fryer and cover with aluminum foil

- In the meantime, coat catfish in flour. Then dip in egg to coat, then in breadcrumbs. Place fish in an air fryer basket and spray with cooking oil.
- Cook for 8 minutes, at 400°F, until cooked through and golden brown.
- Sprinkle with pepper and salt. In the meantime, mix vinegar, dill, relish, mayonnaise, and honey in a bowl. Serve the sauce with fish and green beans.

Nutritional value: per serving: Cal 243| fat 18 g| Carbs 18 g| Protein 33 g

5.5 Roasted Salmon with Fennel Salad

(Prep Time: 15 mints| Cook Time:10 mints| Servings: 4)

Ingredients

- Skinless and center-cut: 4 salmon fillets
- Lemon juice: 1 teaspoon(fresh)
- Parsley: 2 teaspoons(chopped)
- Salt: 1 teaspoon, divided
- Olive oil: 2 tablespoons
- Chopped thyme: 1 teaspoon
- Fennel heads: 4 cups (thinly sliced)
- One clove of minced garlic
- Fresh dill: 2 tablespoons, chopped
- Orange juice: 2 tablespoons(fresh)
- Greek yogurt: 2/3 cup(reduced-fat)

Instructions

- In a bowl, add half teaspoon of salt, parsley, and thyme, mix well. Rub oil over salmon, and sprinkle with thyme mixture.
- Put salmon fillets in the air fryer basket, cook for ten minutes at 350°F.
- In the meantime, mix garlic, fennel, orange juice, yogurt, half tsp. of salt, dill, lemon juice in a bowl.
- Serve with fennel salad.

Nutritional value: per serving: Calories 364|Fat 30g|Protein 38g|Carbohydrate 9g

5.6 Air Fryer Catfish with Cajun seasoning

(Prep Time: 5 mints| Cook Time:20 mints| Servings: 4)

Ingredients

- Cajun seasoning: 3 teaspoons
- Cornmeal: 3/4 cup
- Four catfish fillets

Instructions

- In a zip lock bag, add Cajun seasoning and cornmeal
- Wash and pat Dry the catfish fillets. Add them to the zip lock bag.
- Coat well the fillets with seasoning
- Put catfish fillets in the air fryer. And cook for 15 minutes at 390 F, turn fillets halfway through. To get a golden color on the fillets, cook for more five minutes.
- Serve with lemon wedges and spicy tartar sauce.

Nutritional value: per serving: Cal 324| Fat: 13.9g| |Carbohydrates: 15.6g|Protein: 26.3g

5.7 Air Fryer Sushi Roll

(Prep Time: 1 hour 30 mints| Cook Time:10 mints| Servings: 3)

Ingredients

For the Kale Salad

- Rice vinegar: half teaspoon
- Chopped kale: one and a 1/2 cups
- Garlic powder:1/8 teaspoon
- Sesame seeds: 1 tablespoon
- Toasted sesame oil: 3/4 teaspoon
- Ground ginger: 1/4 teaspoon
- Soy sauce: 3/4 teaspoon
- Sushi Rolls
- Half avocado - sliced
- Cooked Sushi Rice - cooled
- Whole wheat breadcrumbs: half cup
- Sushi: 3 sheets

Instructions

Make the Kale Salad

- In a bowl, add vinegar, garlic powder, kale, soy sauce, sesame oil, and ground ginger. With your hands, mix with sesame seeds and set it aside.

Sushi Rolls

- Lay a sheet of sushi on a flat surface. With damp fingertips, add a tablespoon of rice, and spread it on the sheet. Cover the sheet with rice leaving half-inch space at one end.
- Add kale salad with avocado slices. Roll up the sushi, use water if needed.
- Add the breadcrumbs in a bowl. Coat the sushi roll with Sriracha Mayo, then in breadcrumbs.
- Add the rolls in the air fryer. Cook for ten minutes at 390 F, shake the basket halfway through.
- Take out from the fryer, and let them cool, then cut with a sharp knife.
- Serve with soy sauce.

Nutritional value: per serving: Calories: 369cal| Fat: 13.9g|Carbohydrates: 15g|Protein: 26.3g

5.8 Air Fryer Garlic-Lime Shrimp Kebabs

(Prep Time: 5 mints| Cook Time:18 mints| Servings: 2)

Ingredients

- One lime
- Raw shrimp: 1 cup
- Salt: 1/8 teaspoon
- 1 clove of garlic
- Freshly ground black pepper

Instructions

- In water, let wooden skewers soak for 20 minutes.
- Let the Air fryer preheat to 350F.
- In a bowl, mix shrimp, minced garlic, lime juice, kosher salt, and pepper
- Add shrimp on skewers.
- Place skewers in the air fryer, and cook for 8 minutes. Turn halfway over.

- Top with cilantro and your favorite dip.

Nutritional value: per serving: Calories: 76kcal | Carbohydrates: 4g | Protein: 13g |fat 9 g

5.9 Fish Finger Sandwich

(Prep Time: 10 mints| Cook Time:20 mints| Servings: 3)

Ingredients

- Greek yogurt: 1 tbsp.
- Cod fillets: 4, without skin
- Flour: 2 tbsp.
- Whole-wheat breadcrumbs: 5 tbsp.
- Kosher salt and pepper, to taste
- Capers: 10–12
- Frozen peas: 3/4 cup
- Lemon juice

Instructions

- Let the air fryer preheat.
- Sprinkle kosher salt and pepper on the cod fillets, and coat in flour, then in breadcrumbs
- Spray the fryer basket with oil. Put the cod fillets in the basket.
- Cook for 15 minutes at 200 C.
- In the meantime, cook the peas in boiling water for a few minutes. Take out from the water and blend with Greek yogurt, lemon juice, and capers until well combined.
- On a bun, add cooked fish with pea puree. Add lettuce and tomato.

Nutritional value: per serving: Cal 240| Fat: 12g| Net Carbs: 7g| Protein: 20g

5.10 Healthy Air Fryer Tuna Patties

(Prep Time: 15 mints| Cook Time:10 mints| Servings: 10)

Ingredients

- Whole wheat breadcrumbs: half cup
- Fresh tuna: 4 cups, diced
- Lemon zest
- Lemon juice: 1 Tablespoon
- 1 egg
- Grated parmesan cheese: 3 Tablespoons
- One chopped stalk celery
- Garlic powder: half teaspoon
- Dried herbs: half teaspoon
- Minced onion: 3 Tablespoons
- **Salt**, to taste
- Freshly ground black pepper

Instructions

- In a bowl, add lemon zest, bread crumbs, salt, pepper, celery, eggs, dried herbs, lemon juice, garlic powder, parmesan cheese, and onion. Mix everything. Then add in tuna gently. Shape into patties. If the mixture is too loose, cool in the refrigerator.
- Add air fryer baking paper in the air fryer basket. Spray the baking paper with cooking spray.
- Spray the patties with oil.
- Cook for ten minutes at 360°F. turn the patties halfway over.
- Serve with lemon slices and microgreens.

Nutritional value: per serving: Cal 214| Fat: 15g| Net Carbs: 6g| Protein: 22g

5.11 Crab Cakes

(Prep Time: 10 mints| Cook Time:20 mints| Servings: 6)

Ingredients

- Crab meat: 4 cups
- Two eggs
- Whole wheat bread crumbs: ¼ cup
- Mayonnaise: 2 tablespoons
- Worcestershire sauce: 1 teaspoon
- Old Bay seasoning: 1 and ½ teaspoon
- Dijon mustard: 1 teaspoon
- Freshly ground black pepper to taste
- Green onion: ¼ cup, chopped

Instructions

- In a bowl, add Dijon mustard, Old Bay, eggs, Worcestershire, and mayonnaise mix it well. Then add in the chopped green onion and mix.
- Fold in the crab meat to mayonnaise mix. Then add breadcrumbs, not to over mix.
- Chill the mix in the refrigerator for at least 60 minutes. Then shape into patties.
- Let the air-fryer preheat to 350F. Cook for 10 minutes. Flip the patties halfway through.
- Serve with lemon wedges.

Nutritional value: per serving: Cal 218| Fat: 13 g| Net Carbs: 5.6 g| Protein: 16.7g

5.12 Breaded Air Fried Shrimp with Bang Bang Sauce

(Prep Time: 10 mints| Cook Time:20 mints| Servings: 4)

Ingredients

- **Whole wheat bread crumbs:** 3/4 cup
- Raw shrimp: 4 cups, deveined, peeled
- Flour: half cup
- **Paprika:** one tsp
- **Chicken Seasoning, to taste**
- 2 tbsp. of one egg white
- Kosher salt and pepper to taste

Bang Bang Sauce

- Sweet chili sauce: 1/4 cup
- Plain Greek yogurt: 1/3 cup
- **Sriracha:** 2 tbsp.

Instructions

- Let the Air Fryer preheat to 400 degrees.
- Add the seasonings to shrimp and coat well.
- In three separate bowls, add flour, bread crumbs, and egg whites.
- First coat the shrimp in flour, dab lightly in egg whites, then in the bread crumbs.
- With cooking oil, spray the shrimp.
- Place the shrimps in an air fryer, cook for four minutes, turn the shrimp over, and cook for another four minutes. Serve with micro green and bang bang sauce.

Bang Bang Sauce

- In a small bowl, mix all the ingredients. And serve.

Nutritional value: per serving: 229 calories| total fat 10g | carbohydrates 13g |protein 22g.

5.13 Air Fryer Crispy Fish Sandwich

(Prep Time: 10 mints| Cook Time:10 mints| Servings: 2)

Ingredients

- Cod :2 fillets.
- All-purpose flour: 2 tablespoons
- Pepper: 1/4 teaspoon
- Lemon juice: 1 tablespoon
- Salt: 1/4 teaspoon
- Garlic powder: half teaspoon
- One egg
- Mayo: half tablespoon
- Whole wheat bread crumbs: half cup

Instructions

- In a bowl, add salt, flour, pepper, and garlic powder.
- In a separate bowl, add lemon juice, mayo, and egg.
- In another bowl, add the breadcrumbs.
- Coat the fish in flour, then in egg, then in breadcrumbs.
- With cooking oil, spray the basket and put the fish in the basket. Also, spray the fish with cooking oil.
- Cook at 400 F for ten minutes. This fish is soft, be careful if you flip.

Nutritional Value: per serving: Cal 218| Net Carbs:7g| Fat:12g| Protein: 22g

5.14 Easy Shrimp Egg Rolls

(Prep Time: 20 mints| Cook Time:20 mints| Servings: 6)

Ingredients

- 2-3 cloves of minced garlic
- 12-14 **egg roll wrappers**
- 2-3 cloves of minced garlic
- Raw shrimp (roughly chopped): 4 cups, peeled and deveined
- Coleslaw mix: 3 cups
- **Sesame oil:** 1 and 1/2 teaspoons
- **Soy sauce:** 1 tablespoon
- **Fish sauce:** 1 teaspoon
- Salt, pepper to taste
- **Grated ginger:** half tsp.
- Two green onions chopped
- Water: one cup

Instructions

- In a skillet, add shrimp with garlic, kosher salt, and pepper, spray with cooking oil and sauté until shrimp is pink. Turn off the heat and set it aside.
- In a bowl, add coleslaw mix, cooked shrimp, green onions, fish sauce, soy sauce, sesame oil, and ginger. Mix well.
- Add two tbsp. Of filling, in each wrapper, seal tightly with water.

- With cooking oil, spray the air fryer basket. Place egg rolls in a single layer in the basket. Spray with cooking oil.
- Cook for 7 minutes at 400 degrees. Flip the rolls, then cook for five minutes more.
- Serve with micro green salad.

Nutritional value: per serving: 228 calories| 11g fat| 11g carbs| 20g protein

5.15 Easy Shrimp PO' Boy

(Prep Time: 20 mints| Cook Time:10 mints| Servings: 4)

Ingredients

- Iceberg lettuce: 2 cups shredded
- Shrimp:4 cups, deveined
- Buttermilk: 1/4 cup
- **Fish Fry Coating**: 1/2 cup
- **Creole Seasoning**: 1 teaspoon
- Eight slices of tomato

Remoulade Sauce

- **Creole Seasoning**: half tsp.
- **Mayo**: half cup(reduced-fat)
- Half lemon's juice
- Dijon mustard: 1 tsp
- Worcestershire: 1 tsp
- Minced garlic: one tsp.
- One green onion chopped
- Hot sauce: one tsp

Instructions

Remoulade Sauce

- Mix all ingredients in a bowl. Chill in Refrigerator.

Shrimp

- In a zip lock bag, add buttermilk and Creole seasoning with shrimp and mix well, marinate for half an hour.
- With cooking oil, spray the air fryer basket. Place the shrimp in the air fryer basket.
- Spray the shrimp with olive oil.
- Cook at 400 F for five minutes. Turn the shrimps over, and cook for another five minutes.
- Add the remoulade sauce on whole-wheat bread. Then add tomato slices and lettuce on top, then the shrimp. Enjoy

Nutritional value: per serving: 247 Kcal| total fat 19.3g |carbohydrates 15.6g | protein 24.7g

5.16 Quick & Easy Air Fryer Salmon

(Prep Time: 5 mints| Cook Time:12 mints| Servings: 4)

Ingredients

- **Lemon pepper seasoning**: 2 teaspoons
- Salmon: 4 cups
- **Olive oil**: one tablespoon
- **Seafood seasoning**:2 teaspoons
- Half lemon's juice
- **Garlic powder**:1 teaspoon
- Kosher salt to taste

Instructions

- In a bowl, add one tbsp. of olive oil and half lemon's juice.
- Pour this mixture over salmon and rub. Leave the skin on salmon. It will come off when cooked.
- Rub the salmon with kosher salt and spices.
- Put **parchment paper** in the air fryer basket. Put the salmon in the air fryer.
- Cook at 360 F for ten minutes. Cook until inner salmon temperature reaches 140 F.
- Let the salmon rest five minutes before serving.
- Serve with salad greens and lemon wedges.

Nutritional value: per serving: 132 Cal | total fat 7.4g |carbohydrates 12 g | protein 22.1g

5.17 Air Fryer Parmesan Shrimp

(Prep Time: 5 mints| Cook Time:10 mints| Servings: 4)

Ingredients

- Olive oil: 2 tablespoons
- Jumbo cooked shrimp: 8 cups, peeled, deveined
- Parmesan cheese: 2/3 cup(grated)
- Onion powder: 1 teaspoon
- Pepper: 1 teaspoon
- Four cloves of minced garlic
- Oregano: 1/2 teaspoon
- Basil: 1 teaspoon
- Lemon wedges

Instructions

- Mix parmesan cheese, onion powder, oregano, olive oil, garlic, basil, and pepper in a bowl. Coat the shrimp in this mixture.
- Spray oil on the air fryer basket, put shrimp in it.
- Cook for ten minutes, at 350 F, or until browned.
- Drizzle the lemon on shrimps, before serving with a microgreen salad.

Nutritional value: per serving: Cal 198| Fat: 13 g| Carbs: 5.6 g| Protein: 12.7g

5.18 Air Fryer Lemon Garlic Shrimp

(Prep Time: 5 mints| Cook Time:10 mints| Servings: 2)

Ingredients

- Olive oil: 1 Tbsp.
- Small shrimp: 4 cups, peeled, tails removed
- One lemon juice and zest
- Parsley: 1/4 cup sliced
- Red pepper flakes(crushed): 1 pinch
- Four cloves of grated garlic
- Sea salt: 1/4 teaspoon

Instructions

- Let air fryer heat to 400F
- Mix olive oil, lemon zest, red pepper flakes, shrimp, kosher salt, and garlic in
- a bowl and coat the shrimp well.
- Place shrimps in the air fryer basket, coat with oil spray.

- Cook at 400 F for 8 minutes. Toss the shrimp halfway through
- Serve with lemon slices and parsley.

Nutritional value: per serving: Cal 140| Fat: 18g |Net Carbs: 8g|Protein: 20g

5.19 Air Fryer Shrimp Tacos

(Prep Time: 20 mints| Cook Time:10 mints| Servings: 4)

Ingredients

- Flour tortillas: 12
- Avocado sliced: 1 cup
- Chipotle chili powder: 1 tsp
- Raw jumbo shrimp: 24 pieces, deveined, peeled, without tail
- Smoked paprika: 1/2 tsp
- Salt: 1/4 tsp
- Olive oil: 1 tbsp.
- Green salsa: ½ cup
- Light brown sugar: 1 and 1/2 tsp
- Garlic powder: 1/2 tsp
- Low-fat sour cream: 1/2 cup
- Red onion: 1/2 cup diced

Instructions

- Let the oven preheat to 400 F and spray the air fryer basket with oil spray.
- In a bowl, mix chipotle chili powder, salt, brown sugar, smoked paprika, and garlic powder, mix well
- Pat dry the shrimp, put shrimp in zip lock bag and add the seasonings and toss to coat well
- Place shrimp in air fryer basket in one even layer, cook for four minutes and flip them overcook for four minutes more
- For the sauce, mix sour cream and green salsa.
- Put shrimp in a tortilla, top with sauce, shrimp, red onion, sliced avocado serve with lime wedges.

Nutritional value: per serving: Cal 228| Fat: 18 |carbs: 16 g| Protein: 20 g

5.20 Air Fryer Lemon Pepper Shrimp

(Prep Time: 5 mints| Cook Time:10 mints| Servings: 2)

Ingredients

- Raw shrimp: 1 and 1/2 cup peeled, deveined
- Olive oil: 1/2 tablespoon
- Garlic powder: ¼ tsp
- Lemon pepper: 1 tsp
- Paprika: ¼ tsp
- Juice of one lemon

Instructions

- Let the air fryer preheat to 400 F
- In a bowl, mix lemon pepper, olive oil, paprika, garlic powder, and lemon juice. Mix well. Add shrimps and coat well
- Add shrimps in the air fryer, cook for 6,8 minutes and top with lemon slices and serve

Nutritional value: per serving: Calories 237 |Fat 6g|Carbohydrates 11g|Protein 36g

5.21 Air Fryer Sesame Seeds Fish Fillet

(Prep Time: 10 mints| Cook Time:20 mints| Servings: 2)

Ingredients

- Plain flour: 3 tablespoons
- One egg, beaten
- Five frozen fish fillets

For Coating

- Oil: 2 tablespoons
- Sesame seeds: 1/2 cup
- Rosemary herbs
- 5-6 biscuit's crumbs
- Kosher salt& pepper, to taste

Instructions

- For two-minute sauté the sesame seeds in a pan, without oil. Brown them and set it aside.
- In a plate, mix all coating ingredients
- Place the aluminum foil on the air fryer basket and let it preheat at 200 C.
- First, coat the fish in flour. Then in egg, then in the coating mix.
- Place in the Air fryer. If fillets are frozen, cook for ten min, then turn the fillet and cook for another four minutes.
- If not frozen, then cook for eight minutes and two minutes.

Nutritional value: per serving: Cal 250| Fat: 8g| Net Carbs: 12.4g| Protein: 20g

5.22 Shrimp Scampi

(Prep Time: 5 mints| Cook Time:10 mints| Servings: 2)

Ingredients

- Raw Shrimp: 4 cups
- Lemon Juice: 1 tablespoon
- Chopped fresh basil
- Red Pepper Flakes: 2 teaspoons
- Butter: 2.5 tablespoons
- Chopped chives
- Chicken Stock: 2 tablespoons
- Minced Garlic: 1 tablespoon

Instructions

- Let the air fryer preheat with a metal pan to 330F
- In the hot pan, add garlic, red pepper flakes, and half of the butter. Let it cook for two minutes.
- Add the butter, shrimp, chicken stock, minced garlic, chives, lemon juice, basil in the pan. Let it cook for five minutes. Bathe the shrimp in melted butter.
- Take out from the air fryer and let it rest for one minute.
- Add fresh basil leaves and chives and serve.

Nutritional value: per serving: 287 Kcal |total fat 5.5g |carbohydrates 7.5g | protein 18g

5.23 Air Fried Cajun Salmon

(Prep Time: 10 mints| Cook Time:20 mints| Servings: 1)

Ingredients

- Fresh salmon: 1 piece

- Cajun seasoning: 2 tbsp.
- Lemon juice.

Instructions

- Let the air fryer preheat to 180 C.
- Pat dry the salmon fillet. Rub lemon juice and Cajun seasoning over the fish fillet.
- Place in the air fryer, cook for 7 minutes. Serve with salad greens and lime wedges.

Nutritional value: per serving: 216 Cal | total fat 19g |carbohydrates 5.6g |protein 19.2g

5.24 Air Fryer Salmon with Maple Soy Glaze

(Prep Time: 5 mints| Cook Time:8 mints| Servings: 4)

Ingredients

- Pure maple syrup: 3 tbsp.
- Gluten-free soy sauce: 3 tbsp.
- Sriracha hot sauce: 1 tbsp.
- One clove of minced garlic
- Salmon: 4 fillets, skinless

Instructions

- In a zip lock bag, mix sriracha, maple syrup, garlic, and soy sauce with salmon.
- Mix well and let it marinate for at least half an hour.
- Let the air fryer preheat to 400F. with oil spray the basket
- Take fish out from the marinade, pat dry.
- Put the salmon in the air fryer, cook for 7 to 8 minutes, or longer.
- In the meantime, in a saucepan, add the marinade, let it simmer until reduced to half.
- Add glaze over salmon and serve.

Nutritional value: per serving: Calories 292| Carbohydrates: 12g| Protein: 35g|Fat: 11g|

5.26 Garlic Parmesan Crusted Salmon

(Prep Time: 5 mints| Cook Time:15 mints| Servings: 2)

Ingredients

- Whole wheat breadcrumbs: 1/4 cup
- 4 cups of salmon
- Butter melted: 2 tablespoons
- ¼ tsp of freshly ground black pepper
- Parmesan cheese: 1/4 cup(grated)
- Minced garlic: 2 teaspoons
- Half teaspoon of Italian seasoning

Instructions

- Let the air fryer preheat to 400 F, spray the oil over the air fryer basket.
- Pat dry the salmon. In a bowl, mix Parmesan cheese, Italian seasoning, and breadcrumbs. In another pan, mix melted butter with garlic and add to the breadcrumbs mix. Mix well
- Add kosher salt and freshly ground black pepper to salmon. On top of every salmon piece, add the crust mix and press gently.
- Let the air fryer preheat to 400 F and add salmon in it. Cook until done to your liking.

- Serve hot with vegetable side dishes.

Nutritional value: per serving: Calories 330 |Fat 19g|Carbohydrates 11g|Protein 31g

5.27 Air-Fried Crumbed Fish

(Prep Time: 10 mints| Cook Time:12 mints| Servings: 2)

Ingredients

- Four fish fillets
- Olive oil: 4 tablespoons
- One egg beaten
- Whole wheat breadcrumbs: ¼ cup

Instructions

- Let the air fryer preheat to 180 C.
- In a bowl, mix breadcrumbs with oil. Mix well
- First, coat the fish in the egg mix (egg mix with water) then in the breadcrumb mix. Coat well
- Place in the air fryer, let it cook for 10-12 minutes.
- Serve hot with salad green and lemon.

Nutritional value: per serving: 254 Cal| fat 12.7g|carbohydrates10.2g |protein 15.5g.

5.28 Air Fried Crispy Cod Steak

(Prep Time: 10 mints| Cook Time:10 mints| Servings: 2)

Ingredients

- Two big cod steaks
- Ginger powder: half tsp
- Plum sauce: 1 tbsp.
- Garlic powder: half tsp
- 1/4 cup Kentucky powder
- Turmeric powder: 1/4 tsp
- 1/4 cup corn flour
- Slices of ginger
- Salt, pepper

Instructions

- In a bowl, mix ginger powder, turmeric powder, pepper, garlic powder, and salt. Coat the fish well with spice rub.
- Then dip the fish in corn flour and Kentucky powder mix.
- Spray the oil over fish fillets
- Let the air fryer pre-heat to 180 C.
- Place fish in the air fryer and cook for 15 mines, then at 200C for five minutes.
- In a pan, fry slices of ginger until well browned. Turn off heat and stir in diluted plum sauce, with water.
- Drizzle over fish and serve.

Nutritional value: per serving:219 Cal| total fat 11.8g |carbohydrates 11.1g |protein 22.2g

5.29 Air-Fried Rosemary Garlic Grilled Prawns

(Prep Time: 5 mints| Cook Time:10 mints| Servings: 2)

Ingredients

- Melted butter: 1/2 tbsp.
- Green capsicum: slices
- Eight prawns

- Rosemary leaves
- Kosher salt& freshly ground black pepper
- 3-4 cloves of minced garlic

Instructions

- In a bowl, mix all the ingredients and marinate the prawns in it for at least 60 minutes or more
- Add two prawns and two slices of capsicum on each skewer.
- Let the air fryer preheat to 180 C.
- Cook for 5-6 mints. Then change the temperature to 200 C and cook for another minute.
- Serve with lemon wedges.

Nutritional value: per serving: Cal 194 |Fat: 10g|Carbohydrates: 12g|protein: 26g

5.30 Air-Fried Panko-Crusted Fish Nuggets

(Prep Time: 15 mints| Cook Time:10 mints| Servings: 4)

Ingredients

- Fish fillets in cubes: 2 cups(skinless)
- 1 egg, beaten
- Flour: 5 tablespoons
- Water: 5 tablespoons
- Kosher salt and pepper, to taste
- Breadcrumbs mix
- Smoked paprika: 1 tablespoon
- Whole wheat breadcrumbs: ¼ cup
- Garlic powder: 1 tablespoon

Instructions

- Season the fish cubes with kosher salt and pepper.
- In a bowl, add flour and gradually add water, mixing as you add.
- Then mix in the egg. And keep mixing but do not over mix.
- Coat the cubes in batter then in the breadcrumb mix. Coat well
- Place the cubes in a baking tray and spray with oil.
- Let the air fryer preheat to 200 C.
- Place cubes in the air fryer and cook for 12 minutes or until well cooked and golden brown.
- Serve with salad greens.

Nutritional value: per serving: Cal 184.2|Protein: 19g| Total Fat: 3.3 g| Net Carb: 10g

5.31 Herb & Garlic Fish Fingers

(Prep Time: 10 mints| Cook Time:20 mints| Servings: 4)

Ingredients

- Lemon juice: 2 tbsp.
- Fish: 1 cup
- Salt: half tsp
- Turmeric powder: 1/2 tsp
- Garlic Ginger paste: 1 tsp
- Red chili flakes: half tsp
- One large Egg
- Freshly ground black pepper: half tsp

- All-Purpose Flour: 2 tbsp.
- Whole wheat Bread crumbs: one cup
- Rice Flour: 1 tsp
- Baking soda: 1/4 tsp

Instructions

- In a bowl, add fish fingers, turmeric powder, freshly ground black pepper, red chili flakes, ginger garlic paste, kosher salt, and lemon, mix well
- Keep it aside for ten minutes.
- In another bowl, mix rice flour, all-purpose flour, baking soda, and egg
- Coat the fish in this flour mix, keep it in for ten minutes, and then coat with breadcrumbs.
- Preheat air fryer at 360 F, cook for ten minutes until golden brown and crispy.
- Serve with Tartare sauce and microgreen.

Nutritional value: per serving: Calories 233 |Fat 4g|Carbohydrates 24g|Protein 26g

5.32 Grilled Salmon with Lemon, Soy Sauce

(Prep Time: 10 mints| Cook Time:20 mints| Servings: 4)

Ingredients

- Olive oil: 2 tablespoons
- Two Salmon fillets
- Lemon juice
- Water: 1/3 cup
- Gluten-free soy sauce: 1/3 cup
- Honey: 1/3 cup
- Scallion slices
- Cherry tomato
- Freshly ground black pepper, garlic powder, kosher salt to taste

Instructions

- Season salmon with pepper and salt
- In a bowl, mix honey, soy sauce, lemon juice, water, oil. Add salmon in this marinade and let it rest for least two hours.
- Let the air fryer preheat at 180°C
- Place fish in the air fryer and cook for 8 minutes.
- Move to a dish and top with scallion slices.

Nutritional value: per serving: Cal 211| fat 9g |protein 15g| carbs 4.9g

5.33 Air Fryer Fish and Chips

(Prep Time: 10 mints| Cook Time:35 mints| Servings: 4)

Ingredients

- 4 cups of any fish fillet
- flour: 1/4 cup
- Whole wheat breadcrumbs: one cup
- One egg
- Oil: 2 tbsp.
- Potatoes
- **Salt:** 1 tsp.

Instructions

- Cut the potatoes in fries. Then coat with oil and salt.

- Cook in the air fryer for 20 minutes at 400 F, toss the fries halfway through.
- In the meantime, coat fish in flour, then in the whisked egg, and finally in breadcrumbs mix.
- Place the fish in the air fryer and let it cook at 330F for 15 minutes.
- Flip it halfway through, if needed.
- Serve with tartar sauce and salad green.

Nutritional value: per serving: Calories: 409kcal | Carbohydrates: 44g | Protein: 30g | Fat: 11g |

5.34 Perfect Air Fryer Salmon Fillets

(Prep Time: 5 mints| Cook Time:15 mints| Servings: 2)

Ingredients

- Low-fat Greek yogurt: 1/4 cup
- Two salmon fillets
- Fresh dill: 1 tbsp. (chopped)
- One lemon and lemon juice
- **Garlic powder:** half tsp.
- Kosher salt and pepper

Instructions

- Cut the lemon in slices and lay at the bottom of the air fryer basket.
- Season the salmon with kosher salt and pepper. Put salmon on top of lemons.
- Let it cook at 330 degrees for 15 minutes.
- In the meantime, mix garlic powder, lemon juice, salt, pepper with yogurt and dill.
- Serve the fish with sauce.

Nutritional value: per serving: Calories: 194kcal | Carbohydrates: 6g | Protein: 25g | Fat: 7g

5.35 Air Fryer Lemon Cod

(Prep Time: 5 mints| Cook Time:10 mints| Servings: 1)

Ingredients

- One cod fillet
- Dried parsley
- Kosher salt and pepper, to taste
- Garlic salt
- One lemon

Instructions

- In a bowl, mix all ingredients and coat the fish fillet with spices.
- Slice the lemon and lay at the bottom of the air fryer basket.
- Put spiced fish on top. Cover the fish with lemon slices.
- Cook for ten minutes at 375F, the internal temperature of fish should be 145F.
- Serve with micro green salad.

Nutritional value: per serving: Calories: 101kcal | Carbohydrates: 10g | Protein: 16g | Fat: 1g |

5.36 Crispy Air Fryer Fish

(Prep Time: 10 mints| Cook Time:17 mints| Servings: 4)

Ingredients

- Old bay: 2 tsp

- 4-6, cut in half, Whiting Fish fillets
- Fi ne cornmeal: ¾ cup
- Flour: ¼ cup
- **Paprika:** 1 tsp
- **Garlic powder:** half tsp
- Salt: 1 and ½ tsp
- Freshly ground black pepper: half tsp

Instructions

- In a Zip lock bag, add all ingredients and coat the fish fillets with it.
- Spray oil on the basket of air fryer, and put the fish in it.
- Cook for ten minutes at 400 F. flip fish if necessary and coat with oil spray and cook for another seven-minute.
- Serve with salad green.

Nutritional value: per serving: 254 Kcal | fat 12.7g | carbohydrates8.2g | protein 17.5g.

5.37 Air Fryer Cajun Shrimp Dinner

(Prep Time: 10 mints | Cook Time:20 mints | Servings: 4)

Ingredients

- Peeled, 24 extra-jumbo shrimp
- Olive oil: 2 tablespoons
- Cajun seasoning: 1 tablespoon
- one zucchini, thick slices (half-moons)
- Cooked Turkey: ¼ cup
- Yellow squash, sliced half-moons
- Kosher salt: 1/4 teaspoon

Instructions

- In a bowl, mix the shrimp with Cajun seasoning.
- In another bowl, add zucchini, turkey, salt, squash and coat with oil.
- Let the air fryer preheat to 400F
- Move the shrimp and vegetable mix to the fryer basket and cook for three minutes.
- Serve hot.

Nutritional value: per serving: Calories: 284kcal | Carbohydrates: 8g | Protein: 31 | Fat: 14g

5.38 Basil-Parmesan Crusted Salmon

(Prep Time: 5 mints | Cook Time:15 mints | Servings: 4)

Ingredients

- Grated Parmesan: 3 tablespoons
- Skinless four salmon fillets
- Salt: 1/4 teaspoon
- Freshly ground black pepper
- Low-fat mayonnaise: 3 tablespoons
- Basil leaves, chopped
- Half lemon

Instructions

- Let the air fryer preheat to 400F. Spray the basket with olive oil.
- With salt, pepper, and lemon juice, season the salmon.
- In a bowl, mix two tablespoons of Parmesan cheese with mayonnaise and basil leaves.

- Add this mix and more parmesan on top of salmon and cook for seven minutes or until fully cooked.
- Serve hot.

Nutritional value: per serving: Calories: 289kcal | Carbohydrates: 1.5g | Protein: 30g | Fat: 18.5g

5.39 Air-Grilled Honey-Glazed Salmon

(Prep Time: 10 mints | Cook Time:15 mints | Servings: 2)

Ingredients

- Gluten-free Soy Sauce: 6 tsp
- Salmon Fillets: 2 pcs
- Sweet rice wine: 3 tsp
- Water: 1 tsp
- Honey: 6 tbsp.

Instructions

- In a bowl, mix sweet rice wine, soy sauce, honey, and water.
- Set half of it aside.
- In the half of it, marinate the fish and let it rest for two hours.
- Let the air fryer preheat to 180 C
- Cook the fish for 8 minutes, flip halfway through and cook for another five minutes.
- Baste the salmon with marinade mixture after 3,4 minutes.
- The half of marinade, pour in a saucepan reduce to half, serve with a sauce.

Nutritional value: per serving: calories 254 | carbs 9.9 g | fat 12 g | protein 20 g |

5.40 Air Fryer Crispy Fish Sticks

(Prep Time: 10 mints | Cook Time:15 mints | Serving 4)

Ingredients

- Whitefish such as cod 1 lb.
- Mayonnaise ¼ c
- Dijon mustard 2 tbsp.
- Water 2 tbsp.
- Pork rind 1&1/2 c
- Cajun seasoning ¾ tsp
- Kosher salt& pepper to taste

Instructions

- Spray non-stick cooking spray to the air fryer rack.
- Pat the fish dry & cut into sticks about 1 inch by 2 inches' broad
- Stir together the mayo, mustard, and water in a tiny small dish. Mix the pork rinds & Cajun seasoning into another small container.
- Adding kosher salt& pepper to taste (both pork rinds & seasoning can have a
- decent amount of kosher salt so you can dip a finger to see how salty it is).
- Working for one slice of fish at a time, dip to cover in the mayo mix & then tap off the excess. Dip into the mixture of pork rind, then flip to cover. Place on the rack of an air fryer.

- Set at 400F to Air Fry & bake for 5 minutes, then turn the fish with tongs and bake for another 5 minutes. Serve

Nutritional value: per serving: Cal: 263 | Fat: 16g | Net Carbs: 1g | Protein: 26.4g

5.41 Red Lobsters Coconut Shrimp

(Prep Time: 10 mints | Cook Time:30 mints | Serving 4)

Ingredients

- Pork Rinds: ½ cup (Crushed)
- Jumbo Shrimp:4 cups. (deveined)
- **Coconut Flakes** preferably: ½ cup
- Eggs: two
- Flour of coconut: ½ cup
- Any oil of your choice for frying at least half-inch in pan
- Freshly ground black pepper & kosher salt to taste

Dipping sauce (Pina colada flavor):

- **Powdered Sugar as Substitute:** 2-3 tablespoon
- **Mayonnaise:** 3 tablespoons
- Sour Cream: ½ cup
- **Coconut Extract** or to taste: ¼ tsp
- Coconut Cream: 3 tablespoons
- **Pineapple Flavoring** as much to taste: ¼ tsp
- **Coconut Flakes** preferably unsweetened this is optional: 3 tablespoons

Instructions

Pina Colada (Sauce)

- Mix all the ingredients into a tiny bowl for the Dipping sauce (Pina colada flavor). Combine well, and put in the fridge until ready to serve.

Preparation of Shrimps

- Whip all eggs in a deep bowl, and a small, shallow bowl, add the crushed pork rinds, coconut flour, sea salt, coconut flakes, and freshly ground black pepper.
- Put the shrimp one by one in the mixed eggs for dipping, then in the coconut
- flour blend. Put them on a clean plate or put them on your air fryer's basket.

To Make in Air Fry Oven:

- Place the shrimp battered in a single layer on your air fryer basket. Spritz the shrimp with oil and cook for 8-10 minutes at 360 ° F, flipping them through halfway.

Nutritional value: per serving: Calories 340 | Proteins 25g | Carbs 9g | Fat 16g | Fiber 7g

5.42 Air Fryer Salmon cakes

(Prep Time: 10 mints | Cook Time:10 mints | Serving 2)

Ingredients

- Fresh salmon fillet 8 oz.
- Egg 1
- **Salt** 1/8 tsp
- **Garlic powder** ¼ tsp
- Sliced lemon 1

Instructions

- In the bowl, chop the salmon, add the egg & spices.

- Form tiny cakes. Air fryers preheat to 390. On the bottom of the air fryer bowl, lay sliced lemons—place cakes on top.
- Cook them for seven minutes. Based on your diet preferences, eat with your chosen dip.

Nutritional value: per serving: Kcal: 194, Fat: 9g, Carbs: 1g, Protein: 25g

5.43 California Sushi Rolls Stuffed Avocados

(Prep Time: 10 mints| Cook Time:10 mints| Serving 4)

Ingredients

- Avocados 2
- Softened Cream cheese 2 oz.
- White crabmeat Can 1
- Dried chopped sushi nor, one-sheet
- Finely chopped Cucumber 2 c
- Green onion Chopped 2 tbsp.
- Pickled ginger Chopped 2-3 tbsp.
- Soy sauce Gluten-free ½ tsp
- Rice vinegar 1 tsp
- Sesame oil ¼ tsp
- Sea salt
- Minced Dried onion flakes, 2 tbsp.
- Olive oil, 2 tbsp.
- Optional Sriracha mayonnaise & sesame seeds, for serving

Instructions

- Mash cream cheese with a fork's backside in a medium bowl.
- Add crabmeat, cucumber, nor, green onion, soy sauce, vinegar, pickled ginger, kosher salt& sesame oil.
- Stir, till well combined, using a fork. Scoop half into the avocado. Drizzle the mayonnaise with sriracha.

Nutritional value: per serving: Per serving: Cal: 313, Fat: 24g, Carbs: 12.5g, Protein: 14g

5.44 South West Tortilla Crusted Tilapia Salad

(Prep Time: 15 mints| Cook Time:15 mints| Serving 2)

Ingredients

- Tilapia fillets (Tortilla Crusted)
- Mixed greens: six cups
- Chipotle Lime Dressing: half cup
- Diced red onion: 1/3 cup
- One avocado
- Cherry tomatoes: one cup

Instructions

- On frozen tilapia fillet, spray the olive oil.
- Put in the air fryer basket, cook at 390° for 15-18 minutes.
- In a bowl, add tomatoes, red onion, and half of the greens. Coat with the Chipotle Lime Dressing.
- Serve the fish with vegetables.

Nutritional value: per serving: 260cal| total fat 19g |carbohydrates 7.6g |protein 19.2g

Chapter 6: Optavia Greens & Side Air-fry Recipes

6.1 Salad Green

(Prep Time: 15 mints | Cook Time:0 mints | Serving 8)

Ingredients

- Cucumber: 2 cups, diced
- One Romaine heart
- Green olives: half cup, chopped
- Leafy lettuce: 5 cups
- Red pepper flakes: 1/4 teaspoon
- Cherry tomatoes: half cup

Instructions

- Chop and dice all vegetables. Mix them.
- Add kosher salt and pepper along with chili flakes.
- Drizzle with any Italian dressing, if needed.
- Serve with any lean protein.

Nutritional value: per serving: Total Fat 7g | Total Carbohydrate 2.2 | Protein 1.5G

6.2 Ranch Seasoned Air Fryer Chickpeas

(Prep Time: 5 mints | Cook Time:17 mints | Servings: 8)

Ingredients

- Lemon juice: 1 tablespoon
- One can chickpeas (not rinsed but drained) save the liquid from the can
- Olive oil: 1 tablespoon
- Garlic powder: 2 teaspoons
- Onion powder: 2 teaspoons
- Dried dill: 4 teaspoons
- Sea salt: 3/4 teaspoon

Instructions

- In a bowl, add chickpeas, one tbsp. of its liquid. Air fry for 12 minutes at 400 F.
- Then in a bowl, add fried chickpeas with olive oil, lemon juice, onion powder, dill, salt, garlic powder, coat the chickpeas well
- Put back these chickpeas to the air fryer and cook for five minutes at 350° F
- minutes
- Serve hot or cold.

Nutritional value: per serving: Cal 113.2 | Total Fat2.0 g | Total Carbohydrate 9.1 | Protein 16 g

6.3 Air Fryer Spanakopita Bites

(Prep Time: 10 mints | Cook Time:15 mints | Servings: 4)

Ingredients

- 4 sheets phyllo dough
- Baby spinach leaves: 2 cups
- Grated Parmesan cheese: 2 tablespoons
- Low-fat cottage cheese: 1/4 cup
- Dried oregano: 1 teaspoon
- Feta cheese: 6 tbsp. crumbled

- Water: 2 tablespoons
- One egg white only
- Lemon zest: 1 teaspoon
- Cayenne pepper: 1/8 teaspoon
- Olive oil: 1 tablespoon
- Kosher salt and freshly ground black pepper: 1/4 teaspoon, each

Instructions

- In a pot over high heat, add water and spinach, cook until wilted.
- Drain it and cool for ten minutes. Squeeze out excess moisture.
- In a bowl, mix cottage cheese, Parmesan cheese, oregano, salt, cayenne pepper, egg white, freshly ground black pepper, feta cheese, spinach, and zest. Mix it well or in the food processor.
- Lay one phyllo sheet on a flat surface. Spray with oil. Add the second sheet of phyllo on top—spray oil. Add a total of 4 oiled sheets.
- Form 16 strips from these four oiled sheets. Add one tbsp. Of filling in one strip. Roll it around filling.
- Spray the air fryer basket with oil. Put eight bites in the basket, spray with oil. Cook for 12 minutes at 375°F until crispy and golden brown. Flip halfway through.
- Serve with leaner protein.

Nutritional value: per serving: Calories 82|Fat 4g|Protein 4g|Carbohydrate 7g

6.4 Cheesy Spinach Wontons

(Prep Time: 8 mints| Cook Time:20 mints| Servings: 6)

Ingredients

- Low-fat cream cheese: 1/4 cup, softened
- Wonton wrappers: 16-20
- Baby spinach: 1 and 1/2 cups chopped

Instructions

- In a small bowl, mix spinach and soften cream cheese, mix well
- Lay wonton wrappers on a flat surface, add one tsp of the cream cheese mix in the center
- With the help of water, fold over corners to press the edges together. Give it a wonton shape.
- Cook for six minutes at 400 degrees
- Serve with lean protein.

Nutritional value: per serving: calories 123|fat 10 g| protein 13 g| net Carb 10 g

6.5 Air Fryer Onion Rings

(Prep Time: 105 mints| Cook Time:10 mints| Servings: 4)

Ingredients

- 1 egg whisked
- One large onion
- Whole-wheat breadcrumbs: 1 and 1/2 cup
- Smoked paprika: 1 teaspoon
- Flour: 1 cup

- Garlic powder: 1 teaspoon
- Buttermilk: 1 cup
- Kosher salt and pepper, to taste

Instructions

- Cut the stems of onion. Then cut into half-inch-thick rounds.
- In a bowl, add flour, pepper, garlic powder, smoked paprika, and salt. Then add egg and buttermilk. Mix to combine.
- In another bowl, add the breadcrumbs.
- Coat the onions in buttermilk mix then in breadcrumbs mix.
- Freeze these breaded onions for 15 minutes. Spray the fryer basket with oil
- spray.
- Put onions in the air fryer basket in one single layer. Spray the onion with cooking oil
- Cook at 370 degrees for 10-12 minutes. Flip only, if necessary.
- Serve with lean protein.

Nutritional value: per serving: 205 Kcal |total fat 5.5g |carbohydrates 7.5g | protein 18g

6.6 Air Fryer Delicata Squash

(Prep Time: 5 mints| Cook Time:10 mints| Servings: 2)

Ingredients

- Olive oil: 1/2 Tablespoon
- One delicata squash
- Salt: 1/2 teaspoon
- Rosemary: 1/2 teaspoon

Instructions

- Chop the squash in slices of 1/4 thickness. Discard the seeds.
- In a bowl, add olive oil, salt, rosemary with squash slices. Mix well.
- Cook the squash for ten minutes at 400 F. flip the squash halfway through.
- Make sure it is cooked completely.
- Serve hot with lean protein dish.

Nutritional value: per serving: Cal: 69|Fat: 4g| Carbs: 9g|Protein 1g

6.7 Mac & Cheese Bites

(Prep Time: 20 mints| Cook Time:29 mints| Servings: 36 bites)

Ingredients

- Cheddar cheese: 3/4 cup, shredded
- Cooked mac and cheese cooked with broccoli: for four people
- Broccoli florets: 1 cup
- One egg
- Bacon: 4 slices

Instructions

- Cook the mac and cheese with broccoli, add broccoli in the last few minutes.
- Cook the bacon.
- Then add the cooked crumbled bacon and egg to mac and cheese
- In ramekins or muffin tin, spray with oil.
- Add the mac and cheese to ramekins, top with cheddar cheese
- Place in Air fry, cook for 6-8 minutes, 400 F, or until bites are light brown.

- Serve hot.

Nutritional value: per serving: Cal 258 | Fat: 13 g | Net Carbs: 5.6 g | Protein: 12.7g

6.8 Air Fryer Egg Rolls

(Prep Time: 10 mints | Cook Time:20 mints | Servings: 3)

Ingredients

- Coleslaw mix: half bag
- Half onion
- Salt: 1/2 teaspoon
- Half cups of mushrooms
- Lean ground pork: 2 cups
- One stalk of celery
- Wrappers (egg roll)

Instructions

- Put a skillet over medium flame, add onion and lean ground pork and cook for 5-7 minutes
- Add coleslaw mixture, salt, mushrooms, and celery to skillet and cook for almost five minutes
- Lay egg roll wrapper flat and add filling (1/3 cup), roll it up, seal with water.
- Spray with oil the rolls.
- Put in the air fryer for 6-8 minutes at 400F, flipping once halfway through.
- Serve hot

Nutritional value: per serving: Cal 245 | Fat: 10g | Net Carbs: 9g | Protein: 11g

6.9 Crispy Fried Okra

(Prep Time: 20 mints | Cook Time:10 mints | Servings: 4)

Ingredients

- Water: 1 cup
- Okra: 1.25 cups
- Rice flour: half cup
- Fennel Seeds: 1/2 tsp
- Red chili powder: 1/2 tsp
- Kosher salt:1 tsp
- Semolina: fine,1/4 cup
- Ground Turmeric: 1/2 tsp

Instructions

- Wash and completely dry okra. Slice in half.
- In a bowl, add semolina, fennel seeds, flour, turmeric, chili, salt, powder mix well, and add water to make the batter. It should be should.
- Coat the okra in the batter.
- Place okra slices in the air fryer basket in a single layer. Spray with some oil
- Cook for ten minutes at 330°F.
- Toss the okra, then cook for 2-5 mints, at 350°F or until crispy.
- Serve hot

Nutritional value: per serving: Calories: 151kcal | Carbohydrates: 30g | Protein: 4g | Fat: 1g |

6.10 Baked Sweet Potato Cauliflower Patties

(Prep Time: 15 mints| Cook Time:20 mints| Servings: 7)

Ingredients

- Organic ranch seasoning mix: 2 tbsp.
- One sweet potato
- One diced green onion
- Chili powder: 1/2 tsp
- Minced garlic: 1 tsp
- Packed cilantro: 1 cup
- Cauliflower florets: 2 cup
- Cumin: 1/4 tsp
- Gluten-free flour
- Kosher salt and pepper
- Ground flaxseed: 1/4 cup

Instructions

- Preheat the air fryer at 370 F.
- Peel the sweet potato and cut in bite-size pieces. Pulse in the food processor along with onion, garlic, and cauliflower. Pulse it again.
- Then add flaxseed, cilantro, flour, remaining seasoning, and pulse again until thick batter forms. Make medium thick patties.
- Place them on a baking sheet and put them in the freezer for ten minutes.
- Put them in the air fryer in one layer and cook for 18 minutes or 20.
- Serve with any dipping sauce.

Nutritional value: per serving: Calories: 85 | Fat: 2.9 g | Carbohydrates: 9 g| Protein: 2.7 g

6.11 Air Fryer Falafel

(Prep Time: 10 mints| Cook Time:20 mints| Servings: 6)

Ingredients

- Paprika: 1 teaspoon
- Two cans of chickpeas drained and rinsed
- Cloves of garlic
- One chopped large onion
- Fresh parsley: 1/4 cup
- Gluten-free flour: 3 tablespoons
- Sesame seeds: 2 tablespoons
- Ground cumin: 2 teaspoons
- Cilantro: 1/4 cup
- Juice only: half lemon
- Salt: 1 teaspoon

Instructions

- In a food processor, add sesame seeds, lemon, chickpeas, cumin, garlic, cilantro, shallot, parsley, paprika, salt, and flour. Pulse on high, so everything comes together, but it should not be a smooth paste.
- Make one-inch diameter, tablespoon full balls or form into discs
- Spray olive oil on the air fryer basket and then add the falafel to the basket in one layer and cook for 8 minutes at 350 F. Toss and then cook for six minutes.

- Serve in warm pita bread, with vegetables' slices and your favorite sauce

Nutritional value: per serving: Cal 150| Fat: 8g| Net Carbs: 9g| Protein: 18g

6.12 Zucchini Parmesan Chips

(Prep Time: 10 mints| Cook Time:20 mints| Servings: 6)

Ingredients

- Seasoned, whole wheat Breadcrumbs: ½ cup
- Thinly slices of two zucchinis
- Parmesan Cheese: ½ cup (grated)
- 1 Egg whisked
- Kosher salt and pepper, to taste

Instructions

- Pat dry the zucchini slices, so no moisture remains.
- In a bowl, whisk the egg with a few tsp. of water and salt, pepper. In another bowl, mix the grated cheese, smoked paprika(optional), and breadcrumbs.
- Coat zucchini slices in egg mix then in breadcrumbs. Put all in a rack and spray with olive oil.
- In a single layer, add in the air fryer, and cook for 8 minutes at 350 F. add kosher salt and pepper on top if needed, serve with lean protein.

Nutritional value: per serving: Cal 101|Fat: 8g|Net Carbs: 6g|Protein: 10g

6.13 Lemony Green Beans

(Prep Time: 10 mints| Cook Time:10 mints| Servings: 6)

Ingredients

- Salt, freshly ground black pepper to taste
- Green beans: 4 cups, trimmed
- One lemon
- 1/4 teaspoon oil

Instructions

- Add the green beans in the air fryer basket, top with oil, salt, pepper, and lemon juice.
- Cook for 10-12 minutes at 400 F.
- Serve with a lean protein meal.

Nutritional value: per serving: Cal 58|Fat 9g|Net carbs 5.3 g |Protein 9.0 g

6.14 Air Fryer Roasted Corn

(Prep Time: 10 mints| Cook Time:10 mints| Servings: 4)

Ingredients

- 4 corn ears
- Olive oil: 2 to 3 teaspoons
- Kosher salt and pepper to taste

Instructions

- Clean the corn, wash, and pat dry.
- Fit in the basket of air fryer, cut if need to.
- Top with olive oil, kosher salt, and pepper.
- Cook for ten minutes at 400 F

Nutritional value: per serving: Per serving: Kcal 28|Fat 2g|Net carbs 0 g |Protein 7 g

6.15 Air-Fried Spinach Frittata

(Prep Time: 5 mints| Cook Time:10 mints| Servings: 4)

Ingredients

- 1/3 cup of packed spinach
- One small chopped red onion
- Shredded mozzarella cheese
- Three eggs
- Salt, pepper

Instructions

- Let the air fryer preheat to 180 C
- In a skillet over a medium flame, add oil, onion, cook until translucent, add spinach and sauté until half cooked.
- Beat eggs and season with kosher salt and pepper—mix spinach mixture in it.
- Cook in the air fryer for 8 minutes or until cooked.
- Slice and Serve hot.

Nutritional Value: per serving: Cal 124| Fat: 10.9g|Net Carbs: 14.1g| Protein: 16.9 g

6.16 Pecan Crusted Eggplant Recipe

(Prep Time: 15 mints| Cook Time:8 mints| Servings: 4)

Ingredients

- One eggplant
- Egg replacer: 2 tablespoons
- Whole wheat breadcrumbs: 1 cup
- Marjoram: 1/4 teaspoon
- Kosher salt and pepper: 1/4 teaspoon, each
- Dry mustard: 1/4 teaspoon
- Water: 4 tablespoons
- Pecans: 1/2 cup
- Almond milk: 6 tablespoons

Instructions

- In a bowl, add water, almond milk, and egg replacer, mix and set it aside.
- In a food processor, add 1/4 teaspoon of pepper and kosher salt, marjoram, crumbs, pecans, and mustard. Pulse until well combined and chopped. Do not over mix.
- Let the air fryer preheat to 390 F
- Cut the eggplants into half-inch slices and season with kosher salt and pepper.
- Coat slices in egg mix then in crumbs mix.
- Add coated slices in the air fryer in an even layer—Cook for 6-8 minutes at 390 F.
- Serve with a lean protein meal.

Nutritional value: per serving: Cal 78|Fat 9g|Net carbs 8 g |Protein 9.9 g

6.17 Air Fryer Buffalo Cauliflower

(Prep Time: 5 mints| Cook Time: 10 mints| Servings: 4)

Ingredients

- One egg
- Half head of cauliflower

- Whole wheat breadcrumbs: one cup
- Salt: 1/2 teaspoon
- Garlic powder: 1/2 teaspoon
- One cup of low-fat ranch dressing
- Freshly ground black pepper
- Hot sauce: 1/2 cup

Instructions

- Cut cauliflower into floret. In a bowl, mix the egg with garlic powder, salt, and pepper.
- Coat floret in eggs then in breadcrumbs.
- Add them in the air fryer and cook for 8-10 minutes at 400 F.
- Mix hot sauce with ranch and serve with fried cauliflower.

Nutritional value: per serving: Calories: 94kcal | Carbohydrates: 14g | Protein: 4g | Fat: 2g |

6.18 Air Fryer Avocado Fries

(Prep Time: 10 mints| Cook Time: 10 mints| Servings: 2)

Ingredients

- One avocado
- One egg
- Whole wheat bread crumbs: 1/2 cup
- Salt: 1/2 teaspoon

Instructions

- Avocado should be firm and firm. Cut into wedges.
- In a bowl, beat egg with salt. In another bowl, add the crumbs.
- Coat wedges in egg then in crumbs.
- Air fry them at 400F for 8-10 minutes. Toss halfway through.
- Serve with a lean protein meal.

Nutritional value: per serving: Calories: 251kcal | Carbohydrates: 19g | Protein: 6g | Fat: 17g |

6.19 Air Fryer Sweet Potato Fries

(Prep Time: 5 mints| Cook Time: 8 mints| Servings: 2)

Ingredients

- One sweet potato
- Pinch of kosher salt and freshly ground black pepper
- 1 tsp olive oil

Instructions

- Cut the peeled sweet potato in French fries. Coat with salt, pepper, and oil.
- Cook in the air fryer for 8 minutes, at 400 degrees. Cook potatoes in batches, in single layers.
- Shake once or twice.
- Serve with a leaner protein meal.

Nutritional value: per serving: Calories: 60 | Carbohydrates: 13g | Protein: 1g | fat 6 g

6.20 Air Fryer Frittata

(Prep Time: 3mints| Cook Time: 6 mints| Servings: 2)

Ingredients

- Three eggs
- Kosher salt and pepper to taste
- 1/4 chopped bell pepper

- 2 tbsp. milk
- 1/4 onion, diced
- Two mushrooms
- 1 tbsp. shredded cheese

Instructions

- In a bowl, whisk milk with eggs, pepper, and kosher salt with vegetables.
- Let the air fryer preheat to 400 degrees.
- Pour eggs in the air fryer basket before spraying the basket with olive oil.
- Cook for five minutes, and cheese on top and cook for one minute.
- Serve with tomatoes, avocado, and lean protein.

Nutritional value: per serving: Calories: 162kcal | Carbohydrates: 4g | Protein: 12g | Fat: 10g |

6.21 Air Fryer Kale Chips

(Prep Time: 3 mints| Cook Time: 5 mints| Servings: 2)

Ingredients

- One bunch of kale
- Half tsp. of **garlic powder**
- One tsp. of **olive oil**
- Half tsp. of **salt**

Instructions

- Let the air fryer preheat to 370 degrees.
- Cut the kale in small pieces without the stem.
- In a bowl, add all ingredients with kale pieces.
- Add kale in the air fryer.
- Cook for three minutes. Toss it and cook for two minutes more.
- Serve with a lean protein meal.

Nutritional value: per serving: Calories: 37kcal | Carbohydrates: 6g | Protein: 3g | Fat: 1g |

6.22 Avocado Egg Rolls

(Prep Time: 15mints| Cook Time: 15 mints| Servings: 10)

Ingredients

- Ten egg roll wrappers
- Diced sundried tomatoes: ¼ cup oil drained
- Avocados, cut in cube
- Red onion: 2/3 cup chopped
- 1/3 cup chopped cilantro
- Kosher salt and freshly ground black pepper
- Two small limes: juice

Instructions

- In a bowl, add sundried tomatoes, avocado, cilantro, lime juice, pepper, onion, and kosher salt mix well gently.
- Lay egg roll wrapper flat on a surface, add ¼ cup of filling in the wrapper's bottom.
- Seal with water, and make it into a roll.

- Spray the rolls with olive oil.
- Cook at 400 F in the air fryer for six minutes. Turn halfway through.
- Serve with a leaner protein meal.

Nutritional value: per serving: 160 Cal | total fat 19g | carbohydrates 5.6g | protein 19.2g

6.23 Crispy Air Fryer Brussels Sprouts

(Prep Time: 5 mints | Cook Time: 10 mints | Servings: 4)

Ingredients

- Almonds sliced: 1/4 cup
- Brussel sprouts: 2 cups
- Kosher salt
- Parmesan cheese: 1/4 cup grated
- Olive oil: 2 Tablespoons
- Everything bagel seasoning: 2 Tablespoons

Instructions

- In a saucepan, add Brussel sprouts with two cups of water and let it cook over medium flame for almost ten minutes.
- Drain the sprouts and cut in half.
- In a mixing bowl, add sliced Brussel sprout with crushed almonds, oil, salt, parmesan cheese, and everything bagel seasoning.
- Completely coat the sprouts.
- Cook in the air fryer for 12-15 minutes at 375 F or until light brown.
- Serve with a leaner protein meal.

Nutritional value: per serving: Calories: 155kcal | Carbohydrates: 3g | Protein: 6g | Fat: 3g |

6.24 Vegetable Spring Rolls

(Prep Time: 10 mints | Cook Time: 15 mints | Servings: 4)

Ingredients

- Toasted sesame seeds
- Large carrots – grated
- Spring roll wrappers
- One egg white
- Gluten-free soy sauce, a dash
- Half cabbage: sliced
- Olive oil: 2 tbsp.

Instructions

- In a pan over high flame heat 2 tbsp. of oil and sauté the chopped vegetables. Then add soy sauce. Do not overcook the vegetables.
- Turn off the heat and add toasted sesame seeds.
- Lay spring roll wrappers flat on a surface and add egg white with a brush on

  the sides.
- Add some vegetable mix in the wrapper and fold.
- Spray the spring rolls with oil spray and air dry for 8 minutes at 200 C.
- serve with dipping sauce.

Nutritional value: per serving: 129 calories | fat 16.3g | carbohydrates 8.2g | protein 12.1 g

6.25 Mozzarella Cheese Sticks

(Prep Time: 10 mints| Cook Time: 15 mints| Servings: 4)

Ingredients

- Half-block of mozzarella cheese
- Olive oil
- Powder garlic: 1 tsp
- One egg
- Whole wheat bread crumbs: 1 cup
- Salt: 1/2 tsp

Instructions

- Slice the mozzarella cheese into six strips.
- In a bowl, mix garlic with egg and salt.
- Coat the strips in egg mix then in crumbs.
- Freeze for at least half an hour.
- Spray olive oil on strips.
- Cook for five minutes at 200 C in the air fryer basket.
- Turn every 1.5 minutes to cook fully.
- Serve with a lean protein meal.

Nutritional value: per serving: 224 calories| total fat 15g |carbohydrates 10.3g |protein 9.2g

6.26 Zucchini Gratin

(Prep Time: 10 mints| Cook Time: 15 mints| Servings: 4)

Ingredient

- Olive oil: 1 tablespoon
- Chopped fresh parsley: 1 tablespoon
- Whole wheat bread crumbs: 2 tablespoons
- Medium zucchini
- Freshly ground black pepper & kosher salt to taste
- Grated Parmesan cheese: 4 tablespoons

Instructions

- Let the air fryer preheat to 180C.
- Cut zucchini in half, and a further cut in eight pieces.
- Place pieces in the air fryer, but do not start frying.
- In a bowl, add cheese, freshly ground black pepper, parsley, bread crumbs, and oil. Mix well.
- Add the mixture on top of zucchini. Then cook the pieces for 15 minutes.
- Until light golden brown.

Nutritional value: per serving: 81.7 calories| protein 3.6g carbohydrates 6.1g |fat 5.2g

6.27 Air Fryer Spicy Dill Pickle Fries

(Prep Time: 15 mints| Cook Time: 15 mints| Servings: 12)

Ingredient

- All-purpose flour: 1 cup
- One and a half jars(spears) of spicy dill pickle
- ¼ cup of milk
- Cooking spray
- One egg lightly beaten

- Half teaspoon of paprika
- Whole wheat bread crumbs: 1 cup

Instructions

- Drain the pickles well and pat dry with a paper towel.
- In a bowl, mix paprika and flour. In another bowl, mix whisked egg and milk.
- Put whole wheat bread crumbs in another bowl.
- Let the air fryer preheat to 400 F.
- Coat dill pickle first in flour mixture, after that in egg mix, then in breadcrumbs mix.
- Coat all the dill pickles.
- Add coated dill pickles in one even layer, in the basket of the air fryer.
- Cook for 14 minutes at 400 F
- Flip dill pickles halfway through, until fully cooked

Nutritional value: Per Serving: 79.8 calories| protein 3.1g |carbohydrates 16.8g| fat 1g

6.28 Easy Spring Rolls (Air Fried)

(Prep Time: 20 mints| Cook Time: 24 mints| Servings: 20)

Ingredients

- Asian noodles: ¼ cup
- Sesame oil: 1 tablespoon
- Mince lean pork: one cup
- One chopped onion
- Cloves of minced garlic
- Mixed vegetables: 1 cup
- Gluten-free soy sauce: 1 teaspoon
- One packet of spring rolls
- Cold water: 2 tablespoons

Instructions

- In hot water, soak the Asian noodles till they are tender and then drain the hot water, and cut into smaller pieces, according to your preference.
- In a wok, heat oil till smoking lightly, then add mixed vegetables, the mincemeat, garlic, and onion with soy sauce, cook until the meat is fully cooked.
- Turn off the heat and then add the chopped noodles, until all the juices are absorbed.
- Lay spring roll on a flat surface, one at a time, then add 1/4 cup of filling and fold, seal with the help of water.
- Roll them tightly.
- Let the air fryer preheat to 180 C
- Spray every spring roll with olive oil.
- Place rolls in a single layer and cook for eight minutes at 180 C. or until golden brown.
- Repeat the process until all are cooked.

Nutritional value: Per serving: Cal 153 |Fat: 18g| Net Carbs: 10g| Protein: 20g|

6.29 Easy Air Fryer Zucchini Chips

(Prep Time: 10 mints| Cook Time: 12 mints| Servings: 2)

Ingredients

- Parmesan Cheese: 3 Tbsp.

- Garlic Powder: 1/4 tsp
- Zucchini: 1 Cup (thin slices)
- Corn Starch: 1/4 Cup
- Onion Powder: 1/4 tsp
- Salt: 1/4 tsp
- Whole wheat Bread Crumbs: 1/2 Cup

Instructions

- Let the Air Fryer preheat to 390 F. cut the zucchini into thin slices, like chips.
- In a food processor bowl, mix garlic powder, kosher salt, whole wheat bread crumbs, parmesan cheese, and onion powder.
- Blend into finer pieces.
- Air Fryer Zucchini Chips
- In three separate bowls, add corn starch in one, egg mix in another bowl, and whole wheat breadcrumb mixture in the other bowl.
- Coat zucchini chips into corn starch mix, in egg mix, then coat in whole wheat bread crumbs.
- Spray the air fryer basket with olive oil. Add breaded zucchini chips in a single layer in the air fryer and spray with olive oil.
- Air fry for six minutes at preheated temperature. Cook for another four minutes after turning or until zucchini chips are golden brown.
- Serve with a cooked leaner protein meal.

Nutritional value: Per Serving: 219 calories| total fat 26.9g |carbohydrates 11.2g |protein 14.1g

6.30 Crispy Jicama Fries in Air Fryer

(Prep Time: 15 mints| Cook Time: 15 mints| Servings: 4)

Ingredients

Jicama fries

- Jicama chopped 8 cups
- Olive oil 2 tbsp.
- Garlic powder half tsp
- Cumin 1 tsp
- Sea salt 1 tsp
- Freshly ground black pepper ¼ tsp

Chili topping

- Olive oil 1 tbsp.
- Ground beef ½ lb.
- Diced tomatoes 7.5 oz.
- Chili powder ½ tbsp.
- Cumin ½ tbsp.
- Dried oregano 1 tsp
- Garlic powder ½ tsp
- Sea kosher salt½ tsp

Toppings

- Shredded Cheddar cheese ½ c
- Green chopped onions ¼ c

Instructions

Jicama fries

- Boil into the burner a big pot of water. Add the jicama fries & simmer for 12 to 15 mints, before it is not crunchy anymore.
- If the jicama is no longer crunchy, extract, and pats off.

- Put the fries and the olive oil, garlic powder, cumin, and sea salt in a big cup. Toss to cover.

For an air fryer oven:

- Move the fries in a single layer to 2 racks for air fryer oven. Place the two racks within the air fryer.
- Cook for 10 minutes. Shift the top rack to the lower part and the bottom to top, then bake for another 10 to 15 minutes, until the fries are cooked with gold.

For an air fryer with a basket:

- You may have 2 batches to do. Arrange the fries in the basket, in a single layer, then bake for 20-25 mints. Repeat also on 2nd set.
- Remove racks or basket from the air fryer when fries are finished and adjust the temperature to 400 again.

Chili topping

- When doing so, make the beef chili. Heat the oil in a big saucepan or tiny pot over moderate flame.
- Stir in the ground beef. Increase to medium heat. Cook, splitting apart by a spatula, for around 10 minutes' till browned.
- Put the remaining ingredients of chili into the pan/pot and mix. Cook for 5 minutes, & alter the chili powder to fit (I applied 1/2 tbsp. more).
- Cook, stirring regularly, for about 5 to 10 mints or until flavors grow to your taste for as much as you like.

Assembly

- Move the fries to an 8x8 baking tray or some little oven-safe plate or bowl that works within the fryer oven.
- Let the chili spill over the fries. Sprinkle over with shredded cheese.
- In the center of the air fryer oven (or only in the center of a standard air fryer), put the dish or plate on the rack for around 2 or 3 minutes before the cheese melts. To serve, top with sliced green onions.

Nutritional value: per serving: Cal 216|Fat 3g| |Protein 22g|Carbohydrates 12g

6.31 Smoky Sweet Crunchy Chickpeas

(Prep Time: 10 mints| Cook Time: 10 mints| Servings: 4)

Ingredients

- Water from chickpeas: 2 tablespoons
- Chickpeas: 1 can
- Smoked paprika: 2 teaspoons
- Maple syrup: 1 tablespoon
- Garlic powder: 1 and 1/2 teaspoons
- Half tsp. of sea salt

Instructions

- Do not wash the chickpeas, but rinse them and reserve the water from the can of chickpeas.
- Place the chickpeas in the air fryer basket. Air fry them eight minutes at 390 F
- In the meantime, in a bowl, add maple syrup, kosher salt, garlic powder, two tbsp. of water reserved from cans, smoked paprika. Mix it well.

- Take chickpeas out from the air fryer, coat in the spice mix. Then add coated chickpeas in the air fryer again.
- Cook for another five minutes, at 390 F
- Toss basket, then add back to the fryer for five minutes more, until chickpeas are golden brown and crispy.
- Serve hot and cold with leaner protein.

Nutritional value: Per Serving: 147 Kcal | total fat 19.3g | carbohydrates 15.6g | protein 24.7g

6.32 Air Fryer Bacon-Wrapped Jalapeno Poppers

(Prep Time: 10 mints | Cook Time: 8 mints | Servings: 10)

Ingredients

- Cream cheese: 1/3 cup
- Ten jalapenos
- Thin bacon: 5 strips

Instructions

- Wash and pat dry the jalapenos. Cut them in half and take out the seeds.
- Add the cream cheese in the middle, but do not put too much
- Let the air fryer preheat to 370 F. cut the bacon strips in half.
- Wrap the cream cheese filled jalapenos with slices of bacon.
- Secure with a toothpick.
- Place the wrapped jalapenos in an air fryer, cook at 370 F and cook for 6-8 minutes or until the bacon is crispy.
- Serve hot.

Nutritional value: per serving: Calories: 76kcal | Carbohydrates: 1g | Protein: 2g | Fat: 7g |

6.33 Air Fryer Tofu

(Prep Time: 10 mints | Cook Time: 10 mints | Servings: 4)

Ingredients

- Avocado oil: 1 tablespoon
- Extra firm tofu of 12 oz.
- Cornstarch: 2 teaspoon
- Salt: 1/2 teaspoon
- Onion powder: 1 teaspoon
- Freshly ground black pepper: 1/2 teaspoon
- Garlic powder: 1 teaspoon
- Paprika: 1 teaspoon

Instructions

- **Take the tofu block, and press between** two plates with paper towels in between.
- Add a heavy object on top of it and press for half an hour.
- **Let the air fryer preheat to 390 F**
- **Slice the tofu carefully into half or ¾ inch cubes**
- **Coat tofu cubes in avocado oil than in cornstarch**
- **Coat all pieces of tofu. Then add in the air fryer and cook for five minutes at 390 F.**
- **Or cook to your preference.**
- Serve hot with leaner protein.

Nutritional value: Per Serving: 109 calories| total fat 10g | carbohydrates 3g |protein 14g.

6.34. Asparagus Frittata

(Prep Time: 10 mints| Cook Time: 5 mints| Servings: 2)

Ingredients

- 4 eggs, whisked
- 3 Tablespoons parmesan, grated
- 2 Tablespoons milk
- Salt and black pepper to the taste
- Ten asparagus tips, steamed
- Cooking spray

Instructions

- Mix the eggs with the parmesan, butter, salt, pepper, and whisk well in a pot.
- Heat your air fryer to 400 degrees F and spray with grease.
- Add asparagus, mix the eggs, toss a little, and cook for 5 minutes.
- Split frittata into plates and serve breakfast.
- Enjoy

Nutritional value: per serving: calories 312, fat 5g, fiber 8g, carbs 14g, Protein 2g

6.35 Breakfast Veggie Mix

(Prep time: 10 min| Cook time: 25 min| Servings: 6)

Ingredients

- 1 yellow onion, sliced
- 1 red bell pepper, chopped
- 1 Tablespoon olive oil
- ¼ cup brie, trimmed and cubed
- One and a half cup sourdough bread, cubed
- 8 tbsp. of parmesan, grated
- 8 eggs (white only and 2 yellows)
- 1 Tablespoons mustard
- 2 cups of milk
- Salt and black pepper to the taste

Instructions

- At 350 degrees F, fire up your air fryer, add grease, onion, potato, and bell pepper and cook for 5 minutes.
- Mix the eggs with sugar, salt, pepper, and mustard in a cup, then whisk well.
- Add the bread and brie to the air fryer, add half the mixture of the eggs, and add half the parmesan.
- Add remaining bread and parmesan, toss just a bit and cook for 20 minutes.
- Serve for breakfast and split between dishes.
- Enjoy

Nutritional value: calories 231| fat 5g| fiber 10g|carbs 20g| protein 12g

Conclusion

The Optavia diet's main plan is to help people reduce weight and obesity by controlled portion meals and snacks with low in calories and carbohydrates.

The 5&1 plan limits calories split between six portioned-controlled foods to 800-1,000 calories each day. Although the evidence is mixed, several reports have demonstrated stronger weight reduction of complete or partial meal replacement programs relative to conventional calorie-restricted diets.

The low calorie, low sugar, high protein plan of the Optavia diet includes coaching assistance, which has been proven good, to contribute to short-term weight loss. Its long-term efficacy is uncertain, though. Packaged foods provide convenience.

- Achieves fast weight reduction
- Takes away guesswork about whether to eat
- Offers mutual assistance

The Optavia diet is a series of three plans, two of which concentrate on weight reduction and better at managing weight. The program's foods are lower in calories and carbs and higher in protein to promote weight reduction. Each strategy demands that you consume at least half of your food in the form of Optavia pre-packaged food. Since the menu calls for eating carbs, protein, and healthy fat to be eaten, it is a reasonably healthy diet for healthy food. As far as weight reduction goes, experts agree that Optavia can benefit because its diet is low in calories, for the positive. Still, it's unlikely to change your eating habits significantly. You're likely to regain weight once you quit your diet.

Hence optavia diet has proven to be extremely helpful in controlling and maintaining weight. Still, when optavia lean & green food merges with air frying, it can make this diet much easier for people to follow. Air frying food cuts the cooking time in half and makes the food more nutritious.

You can get many benefits if you follow optavia lean & green air frying recipes along with targeted weight reduction.

Other Advantages

There are additional advantages to the Optavia diet that can improve weight reduction and general health.

Simple to Follow Diet

Since the diet depends primarily on pre-packaged foods, on the 5&1 program, you are only liable for cooking one meal each day. Furthermore, to make things easy to execute, each schedule comes with meal plans and sample meal plans. Although you are expected to prepare 1-3 Lean & Green meals every day, they are quick to create depending on the diet, since the package provides unique recipes and a selection of food choices.

Besides, to supplement lean & green foods, many that are not involved in cooking should purchase prepared meals called "Flavors of Home."

Blood pressure can also be improved

Via weight loss and restricted consumption of sodium, Optavia programs can help improve blood pressure. Optavia can eventually help you lose excess weight. Still, it is in your best interest to develop good-for-your behaviors for long-term results and sticking to a tried-and-tested balanced eating plan like changing your lifestyle for good. If anyone tries to lose weight, it is advised for the long run to care about lifestyle improvements, rather than fast solutions. After all, you're going to have to make those visits to the grocery store for healthy living.

In a nutshell, the Optavia Diet is meant to be followed for short term, and is mainly designed to help people lose weight.

CPSIA information can be obtained
at www.ICGtesting.com
Printed in the USA
LVHW061744291120
672965LV00002B/2